BIOLOGIC REGULATION OF PHYSICAL ACTIVITY

Thomas W. Rowland, MD
Baystate Medical Center
Springfield, Massachusetts

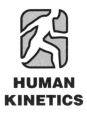

**HUMAN
KINETICS**

Library of Congress Cataloging-in-Publication Data

Names: Rowland, Thomas W., author.
Title: Biologic regulation of physical activity / Thomas W. Rowland.
Description: Champaign, IL : Human Kinetics, [2017] | Includes
  bibliographical references.
Identifiers: LCCN 2015050904 | ISBN 9781492526513 (print)
Subjects: | MESH: Motor Activity--physiology | Brain--physiology | Energy
  Metabolism--physiology
Classification: LCC QP176 | NLM WE 103 | DDC 612.3/9--dc23 LC record available at
http://lccn.loc.gov/2015050904

ISBN: 978-1-4925-2651-3 (print)

The web addresses cited in this text were current as of May 2016, unless otherwise noted.

Senior Acquisitions Editor: Amy N. Tocco; **Developmental Editor:** Katherine Maurer; **Managing Editor:** B. Rego; **Copyeditor:** Joy Hoppenot; **Proofreader:** Jan Feeney; **Indexer:** Dan Connolly; **Permissions Manager:** Dalene Reeder; **Graphic Designer:** Kathleen Boudreau-Fuoss; **Cover Designer:** Keith Blomberg; **Senior Art Manager:** Kelly Hendren; **Illustrations:** © Human Kinetics, unless otherwise noted; **Printer:** Versa Press

Printed in the United States of America   10   9   8   7   6   5   4   3   2   1

The paper in this book is certified under a sustainable forestry program.

Human Kinetics
Website: www.HumanKinetics.com

United States: Human Kinetics
P.O. Box 5076
Champaign, IL 61825-5076
800-747-4457
e-mail: info@hkusa.com

Australia: Human Kinetics
57A Price Avenue
Lower Mitcham, South Australia 5062
08 8372 0999
e-mail: info@hkaustralia.com

Canada: Human Kinetics
475 Devonshire Road Unit 100
Windsor, ON N8Y 2L5
800-465-7301 (in Canada only)
e-mail: info@hkcanada.com

New Zealand: Human Kinetics
P.O. Box 80
Mitcham Shopping Centre, South Australia 5062
0800 222 062
e-mail: info@hknewzealand.com

Europe: Human Kinetics
107 Bradford Road
Stanningley
Leeds LS28 6AT, United Kingdom
+44 (0) 113 255 5665
e-mail: hk@hkeurope.com

Contents

Preface

In the fall of 1999, Professor Robert Malina assigned each student in his kinesiology graduate seminar at Michigan State University the task of writing a critique of an article I had recently published titled "The Biological Basis of Physical Activity" (5). This article addressed the rather provocative but equally intriguing premise that there exists an intrinsic, involuntary governor in the brain that regulates energy expenditure by physical activity in the name of maintenance of energy balance. Presented were lines of evidence derived from numerous genetic and neurophysiologic perspectives as well as a contemplation of the malleability of such a central control and how it might relate to recognized extrinsic, environmental determinants of activity.

So here was, for most of the students, a new and almost counterintuitive concept. The amount that one engages in physical activity is a complex, multifactorial phenomenon, traditionally considered to be established by a mélange of social, cultural, psychological, and environmental influences. Preventive health strategies aimed at improving activity habits have been based on the assumption that such physical activity can be modified by altering these extrinsic sociocultural influences. And, important to this concept, the decision to be physically active or not has traditionally been considered to be just that—an individual's cognitive *decision*.

This article argued for an additional perspective. It provided evidence that a biologic controller, one outside conscious control, should be added to the list of these determinant factors and that this controller has the potential to significantly influence physical activity habits that can favorably affect one's health.

Overall, the comments of the students, kindly provided to me by Professor Malina, could best be described as cautiously skeptical. Here are some samples:

- "If a central nervous system activity center does exist, it is easily overridden."
- "The probability that the human brain controls an individual's levels of physical activity is the latest hypothesis of the human vanity."
- "Wanting to find this biological control and finding it are two fundamentally different enterprises, an observation [the author] has apparently not grasped."
- "The present paper is a good example of a rather new theory that needs to be repeatedly questioned and examined."

- "[The author] severely underestimates the influences society has over both conscious and unconscious cognitions, desires, and motives."

These students found the concept "reasonable," "intriguing," "not surprising," "confusing," "inherently limited," "inconsistent," "unstable," "incoherent," "certainly makes sense," "nothing earth-shattering," "too extreme," and "a little outrageous," one for which "the jury is still out." It would not be unreasonable to expect that such a mixture of reactions might have reflected those of the scientific community at large. After all, wasn't this idea of a brain governor working beneath the level of consciousness to regulate activity, in reality, contrary to common experience? It was difficult to refute the obvious: Doesn't one *decide* to exercise or not, based on cognitive decision making? Whether one takes a walk or sits in front of the television clearly would seem to be up to the individual.

Now, more than 15 years later, the jury is, in fact, still out. And one student who complained that the 1998 article "raised more questions than it provided answers" will probably not be fully assuaged by what he or she reads in the pages that follow here. Still, this time period has witnessed significant developments and lines of thinking that bear importance on this question of involuntary control of one's habits of physical activity.

There is that expectation, based on common sense and each of our own obvious experiences, that participation in regular physical activity reflects a person's willful, cognitive decision making. Well, maybe. But is it possible here that our thinking brains could be deceived on the matter? Some, including neurologist Robert Burton, think so. Writing in *A Skeptic's Guide to the Mind,* Dr. Burton contended that "common sense is merely the strong sense of what is familiar and right, not a truth or guarantee of fact. . . . Feelings about our involuntarily generated subconscious thoughts often feel like deliberate actions of the conscious mind" (1, p. 10). This can happen, since Burton noted that "our brains possess involuntary mechanisms that make unbiased thought impossible yet create the illusion that we are rational creatures capable of fully understanding the mind created by the same mechanisms" (p. 6). That is, we are asking the same conscious mental process to judge whether the mind is being duped or not, as Burton wrote: "Hiring the mind as a consultant for understanding the mind feels like the metaphoric equivalent of asking a known con man for his self-appraisal and letter of reference" (p. 51).

Consistent with this argument, growing evidence suggests that the belief that the conscious mind is firmly in control of human actions and behaviors may be largely a matter of human conceit. Instead it has become increasingly apparent that influences that lie beneath the level of consciousness dictate a great deal of how we conduct our lives. Such an idea, of course, is not new. Arthur Schopenhauer and other philosophers proposed the power of the subconscious more than 200 years ago, Sigmund Freud popularized the concept, and marketing firms now rely on it.

Over the past several decades, particularly with the use of neuroimaging studies, has come increasing evidence that what we once thought was ours to reason and contemplate is, in fact, often strongly influenced by the subconscious mind. How we make decisions (whom to marry, what make of car to buy) appears to be largely dictated by subconscious forces (3). And so it is, as well, with many of the mistakes we make in life (2). The limits of athletic performance, like a marathon race, may be controlled by a subconscious governor in the brain acting to prevent catastrophic injury (without which, it has been argued, one might suffer myocardial damage, coronary insufficiency, muscular tetany, and heatstroke) (7). Electroencephalographic evidence has suggested that the brain can make supposedly cognitive decisions *before* they enter consciousness (4).

Some of these subconscious controllers of behavior have no doubt been installed by sociocultural influences imparted early on in our lives by parents, peers, and teachers. But others are clearly biologic, a product of one's genetic heritage molded by millions of years of Darwinian evolutionary influence. The idea that an involuntary biologic controller of physical activity should exist, then, has gained conceptual credibility, having shifted from being deemed bizarre to being integrated into the current of mainstream thinking.

What has not changed is the recognition of the importance of the issue—the far-reaching role that physical activity habits play in promoting health and well-being. Those who exercise regularly can be expected to experience a decreased risk of infirmities such as coronary artery disease, obesity, hypertension, and stroke. That such diseases represent the principal causes of morbidity and mortality in developed countries lends credence to the importance of such efforts to improve the activity habits of the population. Moreover, in children, who normally do not suffer from such illnesses, evidence continues to grow that early establishment of physical activity habits may lessen the risk of developing such adverse health outcomes in the later adult years (6).

Improving activity habits to salutary ends, then, is a high-priority public health endeavor. To define effective strategies for accomplishing this, the determinant facts that engage us to move around in our daily lives need to be clarified. It is timely in this book, then, to revisit this question of biological control of physical activity and to review the supportive evidence and rationale for its existence, the mechanisms by which it might function, and the implications that such involuntary regulation might carry for interventions to improve habits of regular physical activity.

The chapters that follow develop the concept surrounding a sub-conscious regulator of daily energy expenditure in a linear fashion: evidence ➜ rationale ➜ implications. After a general introduction to the topic, part I presents the diverse evidence, both in animals and humans, that supports the existence of such central control over habitual physical activity. This includes lifetime activity patterns, sex differences in activity, and the effects of experimental brain lesions in animals and disease states in humans. Advances in molecular genetics are described that offer evidence for genetic control of habitual activity in both animals and humans, and the implications of the phenomenon of physical play to biologic control of motor activity are presented.

Part II describes in further detail the possible biologic explanation for control of energy output through activity and proposes a mechanism by which it might function. That central control of physical activity aids in maintaining balance between energy in and energy out seems plausible, particularly as viewed from an aspect of developmental patterns in the various contributors to such balance. The parallels to biologic control of appetite are obvious, and a similar mechanism for activity regulation may be operant.

Part III addresses the most difficult and perhaps most controversial issue: If such a biologic controller of activity exists—and the evidence is quite convincing that, in fact, at least to some extent, it does—so what? Does it play a minor or major role in regulating activity habits? Can it be altered? There are currently many critical questions but few answers. The discussion in part III also reflects on how small derangements in these determinants of energy balance, including motor activity, can be linked to obesity outcomes. This part also examines the intriguing possibility that pharmaceutical agents will be identified that can influence gene action or alter energy balance through motor activity.

This consideration of a biological controller of physical activity embraces a range of domains, from molecular genetics to patients with hyperactivity disorders. It might be anticipated that many readers will need to step outside familiar areas of knowledge to appreciate this multitude of pertinent information. In an effort to facilitate this, the material in this book has been generously referenced, often with citations to review articles.

The chapters in this book are liberally sprinkled with direct quotes from expert witnesses to the issues being considered. Many have weighed in on the question of biological control of physical activity and the factors by which it might be modified.

Throughout this book are frequent allusions to anatomic loci in the central nervous system, which to most will undoubtedly be entirely obscure (the cingulate gyrus, the substantia nigra, and so forth). It has been my well-considered decision to leave such terms undefined rather than provide an extensive tutorial in neuroanatomy. The inclusion of such terms will be useful to those who have knowledge of brain anatomy. If, on the other hand, such terms are foreign, the specific locations of brain function will not be critical to understanding the point that anatomic centers can be identified in certain experimental or clinical situations that have bearing on the question of biologic control of activity.

The thrust of this book is an examination of the validity, rationale, and implications of an intrinsic controller of habitual physical activity as such a governor might operate in healthy, *lean* individuals. It is recognized that the issues of the cause, prevention, and treatment of obesity are closely linked to intrinsic versus extrinsic control of energy expenditure. Still, it would take a separate volume to address the mass of data surrounding the influence of biological control of activity on obesity. Chapter 13 presents a brief excursion into this issue.

Additional caveats should be kept in mind. First, information is generally limited to healthy individuals (except in the case when a particular illness or disease condition might provide insight into basic mechanisms). Second, the influence of sex is largely ignored. Male–female differences in the great majority of the issues in this book have not been adequately studied. The exception is the discussion in chapter 3 of sex influences on habitual physical activity in humans, particularly at very young ages. Third, little consideration is given to potential differences in biologic control of physical activity as it might be influenced by age, athletic training, and physical fitness.

It should be emphasized that it is not my intention in these pages to champion the cause of biological control of physical activity or to serve as an advocate for its importance. Indeed, in the interests of good science—even here in simply reviewing it—I have endeavored to maintain an objective pen. At the same time, however, it is perhaps best to reveal early on my personal biases about where the truth of the matter may lie. It seems to me that the evidence for the existence of some form of involuntary central determinant of daily energy expenditure through physical activity in human beings is compelling and cannot be logically denied. Furthermore, I find it reasonable that the evolutionary explanation for such a brain governor of activity is likely to rest in the maintenance of energy balance. But beyond this, the unanswered questions begin. Still, I cannot help but be intrigued by the possibility that knowledge regarding the influence of biologic control of activity could play an important role in formulating strategies for improving physical activity habits of the population.

I have thus written this book with the goal of raising consciousness regarding the possible existence and function of a central biologic control of physical activity. In particular, it is my hope that such awareness might stimulate further investigations to address the many unresolved questions that remain. Specifically, we need to know how such biologic control might share an 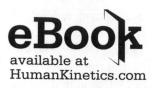 influence over habitual physical activity with environmental factors, and in what proportion, and with what malleability through activity-promoting initiatives. Is biologic control of physical activity in reality only a minor bystander, particularly as one ages? Or does its existence signify a certain futility of attempts to modify activity through environmental manipulation? It is certainly possible, even perhaps likely, that the answers to such questions bear considerable importance in our thinking regarding the exercise–health link and how it might be most effectively and favorably influenced.

Acknowledgments

The many individuals whose ideas and insights have advanced our understanding of biological control of physical activity need to be acknowledged. These include Joe Eisenmann, Alex Rowlands, Claude Bouchard, Theodore Garland, Eric Ravussin, Sjaan Gomersall, A.W. Thorburn, David Thivel, and Terence Wilkin. The courage of these people to challenge convention and innovate thinking inspired the writing of this book.

Introduction

The premise to be weighed in the pages that follow is this: *There exists within the central nervous system an inherent control center that serves to regulate an individual's daily energy expenditure by motor activity.* According to this concept, such an activity governor within the brain is involuntary and acts to influence levels of activity beneath the level of consciousness, differentiating it from motor centers within the cerebral cortex responsible for purposeful muscular activity. This governor is a shared function throughout the animal kingdom. It may act as a means of maintaining the body's energy balance, and its existence is consistent with other feedback regulatory centers in the brain critical to maintaining homeostasis, including controllers of temperature, pH, body fluid content, and blood glucose levels.

The credibility of this concept is strengthened by a considerable body of observational and interventional data from diverse sources in both human and animal models supporting the existence of such an involuntary biologic influence on activity energy expenditure. And, in providing a scientific foundation for such a brain function, that information raises significant questions regarding the quantitative importance and plasticity of a biologic controller in response to extrinsic manipulation.

The role of a deterministic biological control of habitual physical activity needs to be considered in the context of a real-world universal model explaining human motor activity. As depicted schematically in figure I.1, daily physical activity, as with most human behaviors, reflects the causal inputs

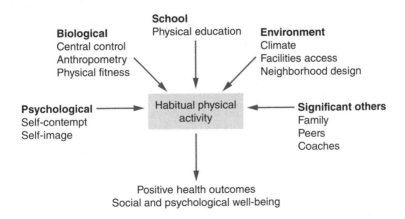

Figure I.1 The basic schema by which multiple determinants might act to dictate physical behavior for health outcomes in humans.

of a variety of physical, psychological, social, and environmental factors. The central argument in the pages that follow holds that (a) such central control exists and (b) its potential influence on activity behaviors should not be ignored.

One of the most compelling pieces of evidence for the existence of biological control of physical activity comes from the observation that levels of daily energy expenditure through physical activity in both humans and animals (adjusted for body size) steadily decline during the course of a lifetime. This fall in daily activity with increasing age is observed in virtually all animal species and is consistent regardless of measurement technique.

As further supporting evidence, experimentally induced lesions in particular parts of the brain in animals can produce reduced or increased levels of physical activity. Changes in physical activity have been observed in human beings with certain brain tumors (i.e., craniopharyngioma). And disease states characterized by increased motor activity (anorexia nervosa, restless legs syndrome, attention deficit hyperactivity disorder) are considered to reflect catecholamine imbalance in the central nervous system. Biochemical effects on the brain that alter habitual activity levels have been described for a variety of administered drugs and chemical agents in both humans and animals. Similarly, certain deficiency and toxic states have been associated with changes in physical activity habits.

If a biologic controller of physical activity exists, activity levels should be expected to demonstrate some evidence of a genetic effect. In fact, from twin and family studies, heritability levels of daily physical activity have been reported to range from 30% to 60%. Recent advances in molecular genetics have permitted identification of specific gene loci that are associated with activity energy expenditure. The observation that spontaneous physical activity demonstrates a temporal rhythmicity expected of biological systems provides further evidence for such an intrinsic central brain controller.

The demonstration that physical activity levels are linked to a level of biological (sexual) development in youth supports a biological influence on regular motor activity. That boys are consistently found to be engaged in greater levels of habitual activity than girls during the pediatric years has traditionally been explained by sociocultural influences. However, such sex differences in motor activity have been documented in very early infancy when the effects of such influences are expected to be minimal, suggesting some biological basis.

AN EVOLUTIONARY BASIS

As every seventh-grade biology student learns, the ability to generate movement is an essential property shared by all members of the animal kingdom.

From the tiniest unicellular organism to the giant mammals of the sea, all have intrinsic mechanisms that transport themselves from one place to another. As a basic, essential characteristic, all animals *move*.

They first moved about 3 billion years ago with a search for a source of energy. At that time, plants, mostly blue-green algae, utilized chlorophyll-like pigments to capture energy from the sun's rays in producing a carbohydrate food source, expelling oxygen into the air as a by-product. For most organisms at the time, this oxygen was a lethal poison, but some developed a means of utilizing this new gas in metabolic pathways that provided energy for survival. The problem now was that since these new aerobic organisms lacked any direct means of using the sun's energy, they could survive only by consuming the energy supply manufactured by plants (as well as by their fellow primitive animals). And that meant they had to first search them out. The obligatory need to track down a food source became the evolutionary stimulus for the development of mechanisms of locomotion (8).

To engage the process of locomotion, the first single-cell members of the animal kingdom probably employed the same mechanisms used by today's unicellular organisms—protein strands that generate force by ratcheting by each other through the action of crossbridges, thereby generating force to shorten (concentric) muscle, push against a stable object (isometric), or contract during lengthening (eccentric). It is intriguing that this basic mechanism is essentially identical to the muscular machinery that is observed when biologists study movement in the current animal kingdom (18). Whether it be the alternative rounding up and lengthening of an amoeba that scoots through the water, the beating of cilia in protozoa, the twisting of a sperm's flagella, or the contractions of complex mammalian musculature, all these actions involve the sliding of protein filaments, one past the other, by a series of ratcheting of cross-linkages. Based on this evidence, then, there appears to have been little innovation in the basic design of the locomotor engine of animals over the course of several millions of years of animal evolution.

What has developed, of course, is the multitude of structural adaptations in designs of animal musculature that have satisfied the demands of running, flying, swimming, and jumping, as well as the changes necessary for accommodating differences in body size (18). Evolutionary developments in muscular action not only have involved means of body transportation but also have provided means for maintaining upright posture as well as opposing thumbs for grasping tools and rotational action at the shoulder for swinging through the trees. Moreover, as contended by Vogel, it can reasonably be suggested that "the ability to make rapid motions was what elicited the evolution of the quick-acting sense organs and the elaborate information processing equipment of animals—that nervous systems, memory, behavior, even emotions arose because we could move" (20, p. 265).

It takes little imagination or argument to explain the evolutionary development of animal locomotor capacity in a Darwinian context. Those who can survive and reproduce most effectively will be those who can escape enemies, obtain food, and adapt to environmental challenges by means of body movement. Moreover, perpetuation of the species will be conferred on those whose mutational alterations provide for the most effective and energy-economical means of doing so. Here, in its most literal form, one has survival of the fittest. And that includes not only capacity for physical performance but also the remarkable plasticity of human neuromuscular function—the ability to get stronger, quicker, or more resistant to fatigue in response to repeated use (for the contemporary reader, that's athletic training).

Indications are that the information in the human genome that evolved to provide these advantages has not changed in the last 10,000 years. But the cultural context of human locomotion has. Early hunter-gatherer ancestors relied largely on endurance fitness (walking, running, tracking), but then with a transition to agriculture and domestication of animals came parallel shifts in more intermittent forms of exercise with emphasis on strength. With the advent of the Industrial Revolution, physical activity as human labor began to wane, a trend that today, accentuated by the Information Revolution, has resulted in the essential disappearance of physical activity—and certainly physical fitness—as a necessary part of daily living (4). As Eaton and colleagues have stated, "humans living today are Stone Age hunter-gatherers displaced through time to a world that differs from that for which our genetic constitution was selected" (5, p. 739).

This book addresses a second evolutionary pressure involving motor activity—the reason or the purpose of a biologic control of physical activity may rest in the need to sustain body energy balance. Maintenance of such balance between energy intake and energy expenditure to sustain a stable body size and composition is a critical homeostatic function. Even small errors in matching these two factors will result in insupportable changes over time.

The energy-in side of the equation—caloric intake—is under biological control from satiety centers linked to energy substrate availability. Daily physical activity and resting metabolic rate serve as the major factors relating to energy out. Since the resting metabolic rate is biologically regulated, it is intuitive to suggest that the amount of physical activity should be similarly manipulated at least to some extent by central biologic factors in the name of establishing body energy balance.

That such a role should serve as the purpose of central control of physical activity is supported by trends of caloric intake, resting metabolic rate, and physical activity that occur over time. In fact, throughout life, and particularly during the childhood and adolescent years, these three factors demonstrate a significant, progressive decline in parallel with each other. Thus, if energy balance is to be maintained over time, the *rate* of decline of each determinant must be precisely matched with the others. Consequently, there must exist a biologic mechanism by which each communicates with the others.

Tight matching of the factors that establish energy balance conferred a survival value to early humans, whose major threat to such balance was a deficit of energy availability. In present society, certain individuals who are susceptible to obesity may suffer from errors on the other side of the equation, when a surfeit of energy source is available. Still, in such cases, the degree of any such daily error in matching of the components of energy balance is exceedingly small.

It is not surprising that the same series of historical revolutions that altered the characteristics and importance of physical fitness in daily living have also shrunk the magnitude of daily energy expenditure as physical activity. Studies based on contemporary hunter-gatherer and agricultural societies suggest that daily activity levels (adjusting for changes in body size) have diminished with each stage of cultural progression (13).

In explaining a central control of physical activity in these terms, one can conclude that the evolutionary process, framed in a Darwinian context, has thus involved two separate key roles for human locomotion—optimization of physical fitness and, as presented in the chapters that follow, control of physical activity. Both initially were an outcome of survival benefits in animals and early hominids. It is not without some irony, then, to note that today they both continue to do so but for altogether different health outcomes.

NATURE OF CENTRAL ACTIVITY CONTROL

A brain center that responds to alterations in the energy in–energy out balance by adjusting levels of physical activity is entirely consistent with the functions of the multitude of the human body's other physiologic feedback controllers that act to maintain homeostasis—a constant *milieu intérieur.* Human survival depends on the finely tuned control of body temperature, acid–base status, electrolyte and fluid composition, and ventilatory function, all of which are established by feedback control centers located within the central nervous system (12).

Although conceptually simple, such feedback centers are, in fact, highly complex. They must receive afferent information input, translate it into a best-case scenario (typically a given set point), and direct efferent commands that accurately sustain a constant-state function. From an evolutionary standpoint, such feedback systems are very old. As witnessed by evidence of biologic control of energy expenditure even in microscopic organisms, this device for presumably establishing energy balance originated millions of years ago. This is in distinction to brain functions developed in the more immediate evolutionary past in which cerebral control acts in a top–down manner, serving to control body functions rather than simply acting in an automatic manner as receptor-responder in the classic feedback system (6). Such function has been suggested, for example, in the form of a central nervous system governor that limits exercise performance as a means of protecting against body damage (16).

The proposed existence of a center that controls amount of daily physical activity should not be confused with the function of those areas of the brain responsible for purposeful or reflex motor activity. There are in fact, multiple areas within the central nervous system that serve to control motor function: Simple reflexes (moving the hand away after touching a hot pan) involve the spinal cord. Balance and coordination centers are found in the cerebellum. Rhythmic movements such as breathing and walking are controlled by centers in the brain stem. And purposeful motion in humans is directed from higher centers in the frontal and prefrontal regions of the cerebral cortex (15).

The anatomic location and neurophysiologic function of an involuntary controller of energy expenditure by physical activity remains to be defined. It is not unlikely, though, that such a center would share characteristics of that of the controller of appetite (i.e., energy intake) since both are primitive feedback controllers that (a) contribute to critical energy balance, (b) involve a physical outcome (activity, eating), and (c) operate as biologic controllers in the guise of apparent voluntary control. The appetite control center is a part of the multicomponent *limbic system* (located in the cingulate gyrus, hippocampus, and amygdaloid body), which functions to organize survival-related behavior, such as feeding, drinking, and reproduction. The key center for appetite, though, resides in the hypothalamus, which serves to organize and relay afferent and efferent information (12). There it recognizes certain biochemical, physical, and hormonal input to identify body energy status and provides appropriate stimuli for caloric consumption. It is reasonable to suggest a similar location and function for a biologic controller of physical activity.

It is not unlikely that such a biologic center would alter energy expenditure by modifying what has been termed *nonexercise activity thermogenesis* (NEAT) (11). Energy expenditure by physical activity can be divided into (a) those voluntary activities that are purposefully designed for improving health or physical fitness and (b) NEAT, or everything else, including "all those activities that render us vibrant, unique and independent beings, such as going to work, playing guitar, toe-tapping and dancing" (11, p. 310). Several studies have, in fact, indicated that manipulation of energy balance can effect responsive changes in NEAT.

This concept of a biologic controller of physical activity is consistent with traditional concepts of energy homeostasis whereby food intake and activity energy expenditure serve as negative feedbacks by which the hypothalamus in the brain sets energy balance to a near zero-sum set point (9, 19). More recently, this schema has been modified to include the actions of biochemical mediators in this process, particularly insulin and leptin.

Not all, however, have been in agreement, contending that the preoc- cupation with energy balance as a homeostatic mechanism has diverted attention away from other factors such as motivation and pleasure that are important in driving human behaviors of feeding and spontaneous physical activity (1). That is, by this argument, factors beyond physiologic feedback can alter energy balance, particularly human motivations, social forces, preferences, and pleasure (so-called hedonistic influences). This stand is based on evidence that activity and eating interventions do not always trigger quantitatively expected reciprocal changes among the contributors of energy balance and that the actions of leptin and insulin (which regulate energy balance in animals) are not reliably observed in humans.

The take on this argument by those convinced of an energy-balance homeostasis model might be that studies of compensations for such altera- tions in the components of energy balance are all short term. Longer dura- tions are necessary for assessing such reciprocal changes, which are likely to demonstrate that homeostatic factors override and compensate for hedonistic behavior. This controversy raises issues both important and interesting regarding the etiology of human obesity: Should excess accumulation of body fat be considered primarily a biological error in the energy balance mechanism? Or, instead, is it an effect of hedonistic behavior involving overindulgence in eating or adoption of a sedentary lifestyle? Or both?

IMPLICATIONS

Traditionally, clinicians, researchers, and public health officials have con- sidered an individual's participation in physical activity to be a conscious, willful endeavor—at least conceptually amenable to change—in response to certain identified environmental factors, also potentially modifiable. For example, Sallis and colleagues reviewed the relationships of 40 variables with physical activity levels of youth in 108 published studies (17). Consistently related variables included opportunities to exercise, parent and peer support, community sports, perceived barriers, and time spent outdoors. Approximately 60% of such associations were found to be statistically significant.

Current strategies for promoting levels of physical activity in the population are based on such premises. It may be a bit troublesome to some, then, to consider that a biologic controller in the brain may play a role in determining level of physical activity, since such intrinsic governors are typically considered largely fixed and resistant to change. Whether this is, in fact, the case for any biologic contribution to control of physical activity is at present unknown. Current information does suggest, however, that such public health strategies for improving activity habits need to be placed in the context of attempts to bend a normally descending activity curve upward over an extended period rather than focus on short-term outcomes. At least one study has indicated the possibility that the biologic curve of progressive decline in activity over the early years can be modified through environmental interventions.

Response to Activity Interventions

The response that might be expected from a biologic governor of physical activity to an activity intervention remains a central but unanswered question. Insights into this issue bear obvious significance to those formulating strategies for improving the physical activities of the population. And, equally important in considering the difficulty in altering activity behaviors in humans is the question of the extent that efforts to manipulate extrinsic environmental factors to improve activity might be expected to be effective in the face of any biologic control.

The response of a central brain controller of physical activity to an exercise intervention might take one or more of several forms. First, the center could act to establish an overall constant amount of physical activity, striving to maintain energy expenditure by such activity over time. As a thermostat works to keep a constant temperature in the room, this *activity-stat* would function to keep physical activity at a particular set point. If a central brain controller of activity worked this way, any effort to increase daily physical activity would be expected to be met by a subsequent compensatory decrease in activity. Some studies seeking to identify such a compensatory decline in activity after an intervention have suggested this possibility, but overall, the results of such observational studies have been mixed. A major difficulty with these types of studies is the unknown factor of the duration over which such compensation might occur.

On the other hand, interventional increases in physical activity could be met with alterations in the other participants in the energy balance equation—particularly resting metabolic rate and caloric intake—to establish a new energy balance that would result in a favorable persistence of increases in physical activity. That is, the activity center might participate in an overall balancing of these determinants, setting the physical activity at an appropriate level considering the other factors.

Here the idea of an activity-stat has a different connotation. In this response, the *primary* set point, analogous to room temperature for the thermostat, is energy in–energy out balance. For this *energy-stat*, the set point is zero, and it adjusts energy expenditure by altering physical activity, basal metabolic rate, and caloric intake at certain levels to achieve this. So here the activity-stat is actually a part of a broader control mechanism (the energy-stat). The set point for this activity-stat would not be fixed but instead would vary according to the status of the other contributors to body energy balance. This concept is not dissimilar to the proposed set point that may defend body composition in obese individuals, one that may create a major challenge to therapeutic interventions. In this process, one would not necessarily expect to observe a compensatory decrease in activity after an activity intervention.

It should be recognized, then, that whether or not compensatory changes can be verified does not necessarily carry any implications about the *existence* of biologic regulation of physical activity. Instead, the importance of such evidence for compensatory changes lies in understanding how such a biologic controller *functions*. At the present time, the functional response of biologic control of activity in the face of alterations in the determinants of energy balance is unknown. Perhaps it is not unlikely that there are differences between individuals in the nature and magnitude of such responses to fluctuations of the contributors to the energy balance equation.

Obesity

The question of biological regulation of physical activity is closely linked to the issue of the etiology and treatment of obesity. Obesity is often considered a behavioral disorder—eating to excess and exercising too little—in a contemporary environment of ready access to cheap high-calorie food and ease of transportation and work without need for physical exertion. If this were the case, however, it would be difficult to explain why *everyone* in such populations is not obese. Indeed, as commonly recognized, some people seem to find it impossible to avoid obesity despite all efforts to do so, while others seem quite impervious to perturbations of food and physical activity, remaining persistently lean.

Normally, the biologic control of energy balance should be expected to closely defend a stable equilibrium between energy intake and energy expenditure. In fact, in healthy people, body weight remains remarkably stable over time, reflecting the influence of a very strict central governor. The obese state, then, can be understood from a biological standpoint as an error—a derangement—in the normally sage regulator of energy balance. It follows, then, that there is an individual susceptibility to such malfunction. It is reasonable to expect that level of caloric expenditure by physical activity would participate in this success or failure of control of energy balance.

Whether or not one becomes overweight when exposed to a milieu of high-calorie mega-portions of fast food and drive-through doughnut shops is an expression of individual variability, one supposed to be dictated on a genetic basis. The subsequent search for genes responsible for common obesity (i.e., beyond those cases involving specific disease states or syndromes) has met with considerable success. At least 50 gene loci have currently been identified that are associated with factors that contribute to the obese state. Evidence exists, as well, that epigenetic factors—agents that determine gene action—act to influence contributors to the obese state.

The specific error in energy balance responsible for excess storage of body fat that would be dictated by one's genetic complement or epigenetic actions remains to be clarified. Alterations in efficiency of metabolic function within the energy balance equation have been sought, but no unifying explanation has been forthcoming. Differences in the temporal and quantitative aspects of compensatory responses to perturbations of energy balance—including level of habitual physical activity—may possibly play a role.

From this viewpoint, obesity is an outcome of three factors: environmental, behavioral, and biological. Such a perspective can bear importance in assessing the most effective routes for preventive and therapeutic interventions. Attempts to alter the march of progress of modern technological societies in providing the ease of effortless transportation and access to appetizing high-calorie foods are unlikely to be successful. The traditional approaches of education, manipulation of the immediate environment, and activity programs to combat obesity are logical, but they have not been met with widespread success. Recognizing the biological basis of obesity may open new opportunities for obesity management, including pharmacological means of altering energy set points and correcting errors in biochemical mediators of energy balance and direct interventions to effect changes in gene function and the epigenetic agents that influence it.

Environmental-Biologic Interactions

With all this information considered, the bottom-line question looms: If biologic regulation of physical activity in human beings exists—and it probably does—what are the implications for those whose previous strategies have focused on altering extrinsic environmental factors with the goal of improving physical activities for health outcomes? Clearly, those factors are important in health-related behaviors; at least theoretically, they are also malleable. One can be convinced to walk to the store for a quart of milk instead of driving or to avoid regular consumption of high-calorie foods. On the other hand, biologic regulators are not expected to exhibit such plasticity—they're largely fixed and generally are expected to be stubborn in their resistance to perturbation.

The relative degree of environmental influence and cognitive choice versus involuntary central regulation of activity and energy balance in physical behaviors then becomes a central, critical question, currently unanswered. One can hope that future research efforts will shed light on this important issue, the answer to which would dictate the most effective preventive and therapeutic efforts at combating sedentary habits. The limited insights currently gained from considerations of compensatory changes to energy imbalance as well as potential means of establishing lifelong habits of exercise suggest, in fact, that interfaces may exist between biological and environmental influences on levels of habitual physical activity. Moreover, such relationships may be expected to manifest a considerable degree of interindividual variability.

Neurophysiological Considerations

The existence of central control of physical activity is consistent with current neurophysiological concepts of how the brain functions. In the past, the brain was considered to work in a responsive fashion, receiving afferent information from the periphery, analyzing it, and sending out efferent commands in response. When an oncoming car veers into your lane, you see it, your brain makes a quick decision, and you pull your vehicle off to the safety of the shoulder.

Now, as German neurophysiologist Andreas Engel wrote, it is argued that there is a need to abandon this classical view of the brain "as a passive, stimulus-driven device that does not actively create meaning by itself" (6, p. 704). Instead, more modern thought sees the brain as an active decision maker in its own right, acting independently, based on experience (both within a given individual's lifetime as well as accumulated during millions of years of evolutionary challenge). In this top–down model of brain function, then, a Darwinian-based advantage is gained by which the brain itself is in charge of initiating body actions—it does not serve simply as a slave to reflex responses in reaction to sensory input from the environment. In this role as an active controller, Engel wrote that the brain "must embody stored predictions that have been acquired both during evolution and through experience-dependent learning, and have proven to be of predictive value" (p. 714).

Here's an example. In the traditional view, a distance runner cognitively selects a pace during a 10K race based on physiological input—how fast she is breathing or how fatigued she feels. That is, it would likely be commonly agreed that how fast to run during the race is a decision-making process by the runner. But some have suggested instead that best pace is controlled by a central governor in the brain, which knows from experience what pace should be selected to permit the runner to cross the finish line at an optimal point, exhausted, without energy to spare (16).

Not all have subscribed to this progressive trend toward a biologic viewpoint of human behavior, arguing that the pendulum has swung too far in a direction that robs the human mind of decision-making capabilities (7). We do not act at the simple dictates of brain nerve cells, they say, but behave within the context of human experience as it interacts with highly complex neurologic systems, ones that are modifiable in response to the events we encounter in our daily lives. Indeed, these neuro-skeptics contend that "brain science promises much and delivers little" (7, p. 86).

Two other opposite—or, at least, contrasting—developments are pertinent to the discussion of biologic control of physical activity in humans. On one hand, the tools of molecular genetics can now provide increasingly specific identification of hereditary factors that affect human behaviors. Such findings are interpreted within the concept of the gene as the fundamental unit, the blueprint, the ultimate controller of human function. In the pages of this book, the identification of gene loci associated with levels of physical activity provide strong evidence for a biologic regulator of activity energy expenditure.

Others have considered this a greatly oversimplistic viewpoint. Denis Noble, for instance, contended in his book *The Music of Life: Biology Beyond the Genome* that this genocentric viewpoint is a delusion (14). "Clearly," he wrote, "the simplistic view that genes 'dictate' the organism and its function is just silly" (14, p. 32). Chromosomal DNA, the repository of gene information, he pointed out, does not act. Instead, the control of expression of genetic information within the DNA molecule lies in the influence of an array of cellular proteins acting in an astounding complexity of interaction, redundancy, and feedback loops, and these can be affected by environmental variables. These are the factors that play the gene. Noble argued for a systems-level perspective, whereby elements at the tissue, whole-organism, and environmental levels can influence gene expression. In the present discussion, this idea clearly opens the door to considerations of interactions between genes and environment that could control levels of physical activity.

For some, these biological perspectives on human behavior have not come too soon. As Byers commented in 1998,

It seems strange that we are just now beginning to study the biology of humans in the same way that biologists have studied other organisms. However, less than 150 years have passed since the publication of *The Origin of Species*, and Darwin's message, as Ernst Mayr (1985) noted, has not yet "fully penetrated" Western consciousness. (2, p. 599)

Philosophical Issues

One would be amiss in this overview by failing to point out that the question of an involuntary biologic controller of physical activity bears significant philosophical overtones. Indeed, this issue might be considered to serve as an ideal model of the basic philosophical dilemma that has troubled thinkers since antiquity: Do humans have a free will to consciously determine their actions? Or are such actions predetermined by subconscious determinants beneath their awareness? Although these issues are clearly beyond the purview of this book, it should be recognized that broader issues besides energy balance and health outcomes are involved in the question of biologic control of physical activity.

Such questions are inherently disturbing. Our sense of security in our lives rests on a sense that we possess *free will,* that we are in control of our destinies. If we are not in control, all is random, and we are vulnerable to fate. *Determinism,* whether it be directed by God, karma, Darwinian evolution, subconscious forces, or biologic governors, eliminates individual conscious choice. By consequence, too, it also absolves us of moral responsibility for our actions, a disturbing sticking point for those who support this concept. That is, if your behavior is predetermined, not a matter of your own free choice, how can you be blamed for social misconduct and crimes committed?

Fortunately, in the question of a deterministic biological regulator of physical activity versus (or in combination with) free choice to participate in physical activities in response to external influences, the issue of whether one bears moral responsibility for one's actions is not as grave as those surrounding heinous crimes. But, still, it does raise the question of free will versus determinism in the context of how a person's behaviors affect the well-being of others (spouse, family, neighbor). In the end, how much is one responsible for one's health? Is there a moral aspect to the choice of using seat belts, seeking immunizations, eating wisely, and exercising regularly? Indeed, it is interesting to note that the entire profession of preventive health is based on the supposition of free will.

As introduced in the preface, at first, consideration of the argument and evidence supporting an involuntary brain controller of daily activity would appear specious. It seems obvious that humans make conscious decisions such as this as a clear-cut matter of free will. We weigh pros and cons and decide what car to buy, whom to marry, where to live. We decide what to order for dessert, what color to paint the living room. That humans (as opposed to animals) have the capacity to *deliberate* has traditionally been considered as the base argument for free will.

There is increasing evidence, however, that much of what we have traditionally considered as being under our thoughtful control may not be so. Indeed, in the age-old philosophical debate surrounding determinism versus free will, the pendulum of evidence has recently decidedly swung toward the former. We consider that humans, as rational beings, make conscious decisions by gathering information, carefully analyzing the pros and cons, and then selecting the optimal choice. Buying stocks, choosing an automobile, selecting a spouse—we assume that intelligent reflection and analysis guide our decisions in life.

Recent neurological imaging techniques, which can pinpoint anatomic portions of the brain responsible for particular thoughts or actions, have indicated, however, that this may often be a false assumption. These investigations confirm that the prefrontal cortex at the front of the brain is responsible for cognitive decision making, for thoughtfully weighing pros and cons. But, surprisingly, the majority of such decisions we make in our daily lives do not arise from this area but instead from deeper brain structures that act beneath the level of consciousness. These centers, such as the amygdala, direct decisions subconsciously based on past experience and primitive emotions (10). The parallels in this story to the question of biological control of physical activity are obvious—the concept is a challenge to free will, a reflection instead of subconscious brain controllers that function as an outcome of evolutionary forces.

The bottom line here is this question: Is the amount that we move around during the course of a day a matter of free will, of conscious decision making, susceptible to modification through education, interventional programs, and manipulation of the environment? Or, is activity energy expenditure deterministic, hard-wired by eons of evolutionary pressures into the brain as an intrinsic, involuntary controller of activity that is largely resistant to extrinsic forces? Or is it a matter, somehow, of both?

It's a rather unique situation—a philosophical question that may be addressed and eventually resolved through scientific evidence. And that underlies the purpose of this book, which is to provide a state-of-the-art analysis of the scientific evidence that has been designed to answer these questions. At the end, with all current evidence and information considered, these queries will be—maintaining their status as a philosophical conundrum—unanswered. But readers may be optimistically reassured that these issues are, in fact, ultimately answerable.

DEFINITIONS

Some definitions are in order. *Physical activity* in these pages is considered in a straightforward manner as the amount that one moves about in the course of daily living. Consequently, it includes any action of contracting skeletal muscle that serves to put the body into motion. It is important, then, to recognize that physical activity is a behavior—it describes how one *acts*—to be distinguished from physical fitness, which is a measure of one's capability in performing a particular physical task. Time spent mowing a lawn is a measure of physical activity. How far one can throw a baseball or how fast one can run 5 kilometers is a matter of physical fitness.

Since muscular activity requires energy, physical activity can be expressed in terms of energy expenditure. Observed activity (e.g., playing basketball) is not always equivalent to energy expended, however, since for any form of motor activity, the actual energy expenditure involved depends on the duration, intensity, and mode of the activity.

As later chapters discuss in greater detail, amount of physical activity can be assessed over a given period by several means. It can be estimated quantitatively by observational scoring systems, diaries or self-report questionnaire, or recordings using portable monitors of counts of steps per day. On the other hand, objective assessment of activity energy expenditure, as kilocalories related to body mass or surface area over time, requires direct or indirect calorimetry (measurement of oxygen uptake) or the doubly labeled water technique. While recognizing these distinctions, the discussions in this book concerning the function of a biological regulator of activity generally describe the expression of this control in terms of *physical activity*, *activity energy expenditure*, and *motor activity*, synonymously.

Besides the variability of measurement techniques, an assessment of physical activity related to any specific determinant is further confounded by the fact that such motor behavior takes various forms, both voluntary and involuntary. Even in animals, where activity behavior should be expected to entirely reflect biologic control, various types of motor activity are observed. In assessing the information provided in this book, then, these issues need to be recognized.

Biologic regulation of levels of habitual physical activity indicates an involuntary physiologic governor within the brain that serves to control levels of activity energy expenditure. The term implies an evolutionary-derived homeostatic mechanism that acts beneath the level of consciousness to maintain activity energy expenditure at a particular level. That any process is dictated by such biological control is evidenced by commonly accepted criteria:

- The process is observed in animals as well as humans. That a process is recognized throughout the evolutionary tree—even to single-cell organisms—speaks to a primitive biological origin.
- Evidence exists for genetic influence (hereditability) of the process.
- The process demonstrates regularity of variability, even in apparently random outcome variables.
- The function and temporal characteristics of the process mimic those of recognized biological phenomena.
- The process is observed to be similar across cultural groups.

You may wish to refer back to these criteria as evidence unfolds for biologic regulation of activity energy expenditure in the discussions that follow.

A proposed biological regulator of levels of physical activity situated in the central nervous system should not be confused with the actions of motor areas of the cerebral cortex that are responsible for dictating voluntary muscular actions (i.e., central command). The former signifies an involuntary controller of total motor activity over time; the latter is confined to muscular acts reflecting cognitive decision making ("I will wave at my friend").

It should be recognized that the regulation of physical activity levels by a brain regulatory center addressed in this book is, in fact, one of several potential biologic controllers of physical activity. For example, genetic influences on factors such as personality, psychological traits (such as self-image), body composition and somatotype, and athletic ability could all have bearing on one's level of daily activity energy expenditure.

A MULTIDISCIPLINARY QUESTION

Carl Craver and Lindley Darden wrote in their excellent book *In Search of Mechanisms*,

> Interfield integration (carried out either during a collaboration between researchers or after hybridization of a single researcher into a multiple specialist) is required in biological sciences in part because of the diversity of constraints on any acceptable description of a mechanism and also due to the fact that researchers in different fields often study different kinds of constraints. (3, p. 162)

That is to say, the mechanisms that might influence habitual physical activity in humans have attracted a large group of very different bedfellows, each examining fundamentally separate issues. Epidemiologists and public health officials are seeking means of understanding how demographic features affect activity and how strategies can be created to improve physical activity habits in the general population. Behavioral psychologists want to know what happens in the mind that drives activity behavior. Physicians seek means of prescribing activity for their patients that will alter activity behavior. Neurophysiologists are looking for insights regarding how bioelectrical processes in the brain affect behavior. Comparative physiologists would like to know if experimental animal models of activity behavior are transferable to humans. Geneticists seek information on the genetic influence on levels of physical activity, and molecular biologists are after insights about what factors might turn on DNA that would direct motor behavior.

This is all just another way of saying that physical activity behavior bears many of the characteristics of a *complex system.* It is *hierarchical,* meaning that it involves processes and systems working at different levels (ranging from human social and environmental interaction to biochemical actions across synapses), has *emergent qualities* (this means that insights regarding the outcome—motor activity—cannot be attained by an understanding of any single one of its determinant factors), displays considerable *redundancy* (duplication or backup factors), and must be understood in *temporal* and dynamic terms (influences on activity exist in the context of time).

Looking at the list of those niches of subspecialty interest that share a quest for insights into activity behavior, this is obviously a mixture of people who do not occupy the same office space (and presumably don't even work in the same building). They need to be sharing coffee more often. Progress in understanding the determinants of activity is likely to be limited unless collaboration occurs among those interested in all the separate levels of this complex phenomenon.

Surveying the Evidence

Numerous observations derived from a variety of sources have provided abundant evidence for the existence and function of a biologic regulation of daily physical activity. Taken collectively, such information provides a persuasive argument for the existence of at least some degree of central involuntary control of energy expenditure through daily motor activity.

Part I examines these data in detail. What is perhaps most striking about this information is the diversity of evidence, including epidemiologic studies in twins, animal brain decortication experiments, and compulsive exercise behavior in patients with anorexia nervosa. Much of these data are derived from animal studies, performed largely in rodents, and the extent that findings in such reports can be reliably transferred to humans is always open to question. Still, there is sufficient evidence that strongly suggests that human beings share similar biologic control of physical activity with lower species in the evolutionary tree.

Nature of Physical Activity

T he outcomes of research studies described in the following chapters need to be considered within the context of the limitations by which levels of habitual physical activity can be characterized and quantified. A variety of methodologies have been employed to this end, but there unfortunately exists no single ideal technique (a) that is not intrusive to inhibit normal activity and (b) that accurately examines activity over extended periods that reflect habitual activity in free-living individuals (155).

MEASURING PHYSICAL ACTIVITY

The contraction of skeletal muscle to produce body movement involves the conversion of chemical energy (in stored carbohydrate and fat) to mechanical energy (to drive the sliding of actin and myosin filaments in muscle cells). The work accomplished by such muscular contractions generates heat, which (quantified as joules or kilocalories) provides an indication of the amount of energy expended in the work accomplished. This increase in heat production can be measured in a metabolic chamber or room specially designed for accurately recording changes in ambient temperature (direct calorimetry), and such devices have been used to examine energy equivalents of motor activity (158). However, this approach is clearly impractical for assessing energy expenditure by activity in free-living individuals over time.

Two other techniques, the doubly labeled water method and the measurement of oxygen uptake by indirect calorimetry, have been considered as criterion measures of activity energy expenditure. With the doubly labeled water method, subjects ingest two safe, naturally occurring isotopes that are excreted in the urine over time. Total carbon dioxide production over this period from the relative elimination rates of the two isotopes on analysis of urine provides an indication of total energy expenditure over 1 to 4 weeks. This method is expensive, and, as an indicator of total energy expenditure (TEE), it cannot provide a breakdown of the relative contributions of its components (basal metabolic rate, energy expended in the digestion of food [diet-induced thermogenesis], and physical activity). When this technique has been used to determine physical activity energy expenditure (AEE), basal metabolic rate (BMR) is determined by indirect calorimetry and dietary energy expenditure is considered to represent 10% of TEE, and AEE can be calculated as AEE = 0.9 (TEE − BMR).

The amount of oxygen ($\dot{V}O_2$) utilized in cellular metabolic processes during physical work (indirect calorimetry), analyzed in terms of gas concentrations in exhaled air, provides an accurate measure of energy expenditure. Although the equipment required for such measures has recently been miniaturized to permit ambulatory determinations, such an approach remains largely impractical for assessing free-living energy expenditure. Instead, approaches for measuring amount of physical activity (such as direct observation, activity diaries, questionnaires, and 24-hour heart rate recordings) can be calibrated against $\dot{V}O_2$ in laboratory or ambulatory settings to provide an estimate of actual energy expenditure. That is, specific types of activities (i.e., walking) can be related to particular levels of $\dot{V}O_2$, or heart rate–$\dot{V}O_2$ regression equations can be developed during exercise testing. Some of these studies have expressed activity level in terms of metabolic equivalents (METs), or multiples of resting energy expenditure (i.e., a two-MET activity involves a level of energy expenditure twice that of the subject at rest).

Portable activity monitors (pedometers, accelerometers) provide information regarding physical activity as *counts*, which relate to amount of physical activity over a period of time. Equations have been developed for converting counts to measures of energy expenditure, but their validity remains uncertain, particularly in youth (105).

Each of these measurement techniques bears certain advantages and disadvantages when assessing energy expenditure from physical activity (see ref. 55 for review). In general, an inverse relationship exists between the ease and feasibility of a particular technique and its accuracy in estimating level of activity (figure 1.1). That is, energy expenditure measures determined in a room calorimeter are highly precise but clearly impractical for examining activity levels in free living in groups of individuals over time. On the other hand, pencil-and-paper questionnaires are inexpensive, simple to administer, and useful for large groups of subjects but lack accuracy in defining activity-related energy expenditure.

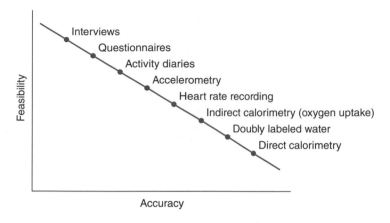

Figure 1.1   The inverse relationship between the feasibility and accuracy of methods for assessing levels of habitual physical activity in free-living populations.

CATEGORIZING PHYSICAL ACTIVITY

As noted previously, total energy expenditure can be divided into contributions by basal metabolic rate, thermic effect of food, and physical activity. The relative contributions of each obviously vary considerably, both over time and from individual to individual. In a sedentary human, basal metabolic rate accounts for about 65% of total daily energy expenditure, thermic effect of food for 10%, and physical activity for 25%. When competing in the Tour de France, on the other hand, the values for a typical cyclist are 25%, 10%, and 65%, respectively (57, 129) (figure 1.2).

Physical activity in human beings can be categorized in a number of ways. *Spontaneous physical activity* includes those minor motor actions that occur during daily living without conscious thinking, such as fidgeting, standing, holding a book, and walking about the house. Such activities are expressed as actual energy expenditure under the classification of *nonexercise activity thermogenesis*, or NEAT (85). Despite disagreement among some authors about which activities should be actually included under these terms, in this book *spontaneous activity* and *NEAT* are used synonymously.

Voluntary physical activities are those that are planned and purposeful, including energy expenditures such as leisure (recreational) pursuits, occupational work, and athletic training. Clearly, marked interindividual differences can be expected in the relative contributions of each to daily activity energy expenditure. Also, variations in voluntary activities are likely to occur in response to temporal, geographical, and climatic influences (100). Adding to the variability in published reports, it is evident that

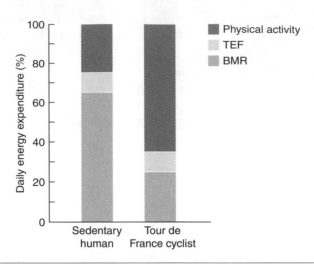

Figure 1.2   Relative contributions of the major factors responsible for energy expenditure in the sedentary human and cyclists in the Tour de France.

Data from Garland et al. 2011; Saris et al. 1989.

not all forms of physical activity will be captured by all activity assessment methods. For example, most questionnaire and diary approaches concentrate on quantifying leisure-time activities and level of participation in organized sports, missing contributions to energy expenditure by spontaneous activity altogether.

Even the energy expended during performance of common activities can be highly variable. Pfeiffer and colleagues measured energy expenditure by indirect calorimetry for 10 activities in adolescent girls (113). Depending on the means by which energy expenditure was related, coefficients of variation were high, ranging from 13% while climbing stairs to 38% while playing a computer game.

Physical Activity Through the Life Span

Among the most compelling pieces of evidence for a biologic controller of daily physical activity is the consistent observation that energy expenditure in the form of motor activity, when adjusted for body size, steadily declines over the course of the life span (11, 141, 146). Not all have been in agreement, however, that this decrease in physical activity with increasing age requires a biological explanation. It has been suggested instead, for example, that "observed age-related differences in physical activity are the result of complex changes in psychological and social factors that occur with age" (70, p. 41). For some health professionals, in fact, this fall in physical activity, particularly during the childhood and adolescent years, has been viewed with grave concern as an indication of increasing sedentary habits of young persons in response to environmental influences—with potential adverse health outcomes (28).

However, that such trends basically reflect a normal biological phenomenon rather than simply the influence of environmental or cultural factors is evidenced by very similar patterns and magnitudes of decreases in activity with age that are consistently observed throughout the animal kingdom. In addition, as is discussed later, the fall in physical activity with age closely parallels similar declines in size-relative basal or resting metabolic rate and daily caloric intake, both recognized expressions of biologic regulation.

This conclusion does not preclude the expectation that extrinsic environmental factors, those traditionally considered as influencing physical activity levels, might in fact play important roles in defining the decline of physical activity with age. In fact, reasons clearly exist to expect that certain extrinsic age-related influences might alter physical activity levels with age. For instance, psychosocial issues that arise during adolescence may strongly alter activity habits: "The motivation for physical activity for the typical adolescent, no longer a biological issue, is shaped by factors that involve peer acceptance, physical capabilities, sexual attractiveness, and self concept" (122, p. 3). Likewise, chronic illness and physical infirmities, as well as the normal decline in physical fitness, could be expected to depress activity levels in the elderly. The information demonstrated in this chapter does, however, imply that any such determinants are played out against a downward trend of habitual physical activity that represents a normal biological phenomenon.

HUMAN BEINGS

From almost the age when they first become fully ambulatory, humans demonstrate a progressive decline in energy expenditure by motor activity (adjusted for body size), a trend that persists throughout life to senescence. No single study has described this pattern in its entirety. However, the continuity of the curve of decline in physical activity over the life span can be readily realized by a synthesis of the findings of multiple investigations within particular age groups.

Such investigations are not without their weaknesses. For example, few of these studies have assessed actual energy expenditure either by equating activities to oxygen uptake as an indirect measure of energy expenditure or by using the doubly labeled water technique. Also, most are based on assessments of levels of leisure-time activity and sports play, thereby ignoring energy expenditure involved in minor motor activities (standing, taking stairs, playing musical instruments, performing household chores). Collectively, these latter activities may constitute a significant portion of daily energy expenditure through physical activity. Based on animal studies, it is not unlikely, too, that such activities are those principally under control of biologic regulation.

These issues notwithstanding, a true decline in physical activity with age is evidenced by the consistency with which a fall in physical activity with age has been verified by all available assessment methodologies. This trend is consistent, too, with common experience. One need only compare the energy levels observed at a birthday party of 4-year-olds with that of a group of young adults to be so convinced.

Youth

Information regarding trends of energy expenditure through physical activity during early childhood comes from the cross-sectional data accumulated by

Turin (146). In 22 international studies comprising 483 boys and 657 girls between the ages of 1 and 18 years, absolute total daily energy expenditure estimated by the doubly labeled water method increased linearly with age in boys. When expressed relative to body mass, a progressive decline was observed, from an average of 83 kcal·kg⁻¹·d⁻¹ to 48 kcal·kg⁻¹·d⁻¹ over the 17 years (figure 2.1). Similar trends were observed in female subjects, and findings were almost identical in investigations that used heart rate monitoring (calibrated against oxygen uptake).

Based on previously published data on basal metabolic rate (BMR) with age, the decrease in mass-relative total energy expenditure with age beginning

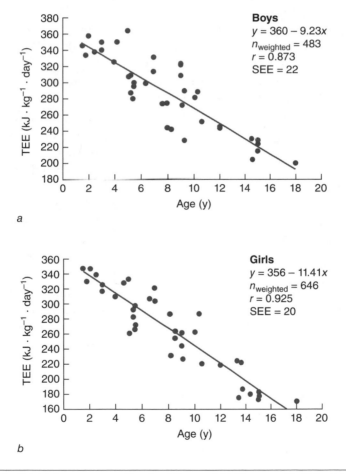

Figure 2.1   Total daily energy expenditure for *(a)* boys and *(b)* girls expressed relative to body weight in children and adolescents aged 2 to 18 measured by the doubly labeled water technique.

B. Torun, "Energy requirements of children and adolescents," *Public Health and Nutrition* 8: 968-993, 2005, reproduced with permission.

in early infancy can be accounted for approximately equally by a decline in BMR and fall in activity energy expenditure (both expressed as per kg of body mass). Between the ages of 2 and 18 years, the decline in activity in boys in a compilation of cross-sectional studies was approximately 35% (95).

In an earlier report, Black and colleagues performed a similar analysis of studies executed using the doubly labeled water method and measuring basal metabolic rate (12). Subtraction of BMR from values of total energy expenditure yielded an estimate of activity energy expenditure (which still included the contribution of thermogenesis of eating). Between the ages of 1 and 17 years, mass-relative AEE in the males fell from 0.105 to 0.065 $MJ \cdot kg^{-1} \cdot d^{-1}$ (−38%), while in the females, values declined from 0.110 to 0.83 $MJ \cdot kg^{-1} \cdot d^{-1}$ (−25%).

Longitudinal studies confirm that the most precipitous rate of decline of energy expenditure by physical activity occurs during the childhood years. Figure 2.2 depicts a descending curve of estimated daily energy expenditure in kcal per kg of body mass constructed from the reports of Saris and others (128) and Verschuur and Kemper (148). The former study was composed of 406 Dutch children who had yearly assessments of physical activity over a period of 6 years beginning at age 6. Energy expenditure was estimated by individualized 24-hour heart rate–$\dot{V}O_2$ regression equations. Verschuur and Kemper used a similar approach in assessing energy expenditure longitudinally in another set of Dutch youth between the ages of 13 and 17 years. These data suggest a reduction in mass-specific caloric expenditure through motor activity approaching 50% over a period of 10 years as children and adolescents grow.

McMurray and colleagues reported longitudinal physical activity levels in 791 boys and girls between the ages of 8 and 16 years (101). Activity scores calculated from questionnaire data demonstrated a decrease by approximately 50% over the testing period, with similar declines in males and females as well as Caucasians and African Americans. In the preceding studies of youth, the rate of decline of activity among males and females appears to be similar, but others have shown inconsistent (and unexplained) sex-related differences, particularly at certain age groups (126).

In the NHLBI Growth and Health Study, 2,379 black and white girls were assessed serially for 10 years beginning at age 9 or 10 years (74). From baseline to year 10, levels of physical activity assessed by a 3-day diary fell by 35% and by 83% when habitual activity was sought by questionnaire. An ambulatory activity monitor employed between years 3 and 5 indicated a 22% fall in activity.

Dumuth and colleagues compiled data from 26 published studies that examined longitudinal changes in physical activity, mostly by questionnaire

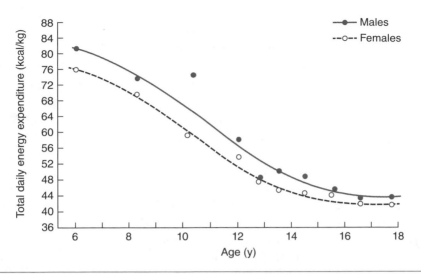

Figure 2.2   Daily energy expenditure (related to body mass) through physical activity in youth 6 to 18 years.

Reprinted, by permission, from T.W. Rowland, 1990, *Exercise and children's health* (Champaign, IL: Human Kinetics), 35. Data from Saris et al. 1986; Verschuur and Kemper 1985.

(41). Included were those reports that performed at least two activity assessments between the ages of 10 and 19 years or included a first measurement in childhood and the second in the teen years. In these combined data, a progressive decline in activity was observed, with an average of 7.0% decrease per year (95% confidence limits: −8.8% to −5.2%). These authors made the important observation that interventions for improving health-related activity habits during the teen years would be considered successful if this rate of decline were attenuated or eliminated rather than attempting to actually increase levels of activity over time.

Any decrease in observed physical activity during the pediatric years is not simply an expression of any developmental changes in muscle energy efficiency or exercise economy on weight-bearing exercise. Rowland and others demonstrated that levels of energy expenditure relative to progressive workloads on a cycle ergometer were similar in prepubertal boys and college-aged men (124). This finding suggests that metabolic factors such as fraction of energy released from adenosine triphosphate (phosphorylative coupling) or percentage of energy used by the muscle to create external work (contraction coupling) are not influenced by normal development and maturation. Similarly, when children perform weight-bearing exercise tasks (running, walking) that are properly adjusted for body size, no differences in *exercise economy* ($\dot{V}O_2$ per kg) are observed when compared to that of adults (123).

Adulthood

Several studies have examined longitudinal changes in levels of physical activity spanning the years from adolescence to mid-adulthood. In the Amsterdam Longitudinal Growth and Health Study, 181 males and females completed a series of six assessments between the ages of 13 and 27 years (147). Amount of physical activity in the previous 3 months was determined by an interview-administered questionnaire that sought information quantifying time spent in activities at school, work, and sports as well as in other leisure-time activities. These data were converted to estimated energy expenditure as estimated metabolic equivalents (METs). Between the ages of 13 and 27 years, average physical activity level fell from 4,990 to 2,910 METs per week in the males (−42%) and from 3,810 to 3,180 METs weekly in the females (−17%). Declines in time per week in activities >4 METs were −31% and −8% in the two groups, respectively, over the 15-year study period. Highest rates of fall in activity in METs per week occurred during the early adolescent period up to age 16 years.

These findings mimicked those of the Cardiovascular Risk in Young Finns project, which assessed participation in physical activities serially between the ages of 9 and 27 years (141). A short questionnaire sought information regarding frequency and intensity of leisure-time activities, participation in competitive sports, and means of spending leisure time. Activity was scored by an index (there was no conversion to estimated energy expenditure). Self-reported physical activity fell during the study period by 57% in males and 28% in females.

Caspersen and colleagues provided cross-sectional data from two large-scale investigations of physical activity of subjects aged 12 and up (some more than 75 years old) (27). Participation in leisure-time activities was sought by questionnaire. The trend in the 12-to-21 age group showed a decline in sustained activities of 6% in the males and 10% in females, while time in vigorous activities declined over the same period by 29% and 36%, respectively. In the adults the decrease was less abrupt, with a decline of 7% in regular sustained exercise in males between young adulthood (18-29) and age 75, while the females showed a 9% decrease. Interestingly, however, increases of 19% and 6%, respectively, were described in regular vigorous activities between age groups 18 to 29 and 75 years.

Old Age

Longitudinal investigations confirm that the lifelong trend for decreasing mass-specific energy expenditure by physical activity persists through the elderly years (135). For example, Bijnen and colleagues described changes in self-reported physical activity in 343 Dutch men aged 65 to 84 years over a 10-year period (1985-1995) (11). Average total time spent participating in physical activities during this period fell by 33%. The authors concluded that this trend was not explained by deterioration in functional status.

In a cross-sectional study, Starling and others found an inverse relationship between chronological age and physical activity energy expenditure (kcal/d) in women aged 52 to 85 years using doubly labeled water and indirect calorimetry ($r = -0.44$) (136) (figure 2.3). A similar investigation in elderly men mimicked these findings, with a negative correlation between age and activity energy expenditure ($r = -0.36$) (119).

Considering the different methodologies and definitions employed in directly assessing activity, it is difficult to compare these life-span studies. The various individual types and levels of activities in a number of these reports change over time, and certain forms of exercise may be sex-specific (i.e., males may be more involved in organized sports during adolescence) (95). Nonetheless, despite the pitfalls of measurement techniques, varying populations, types and intensity of activities assessed, sex-related differences, and inter- and intraindividual variability, the consistency of the findings of a pronounced, progressive decline of overall level of daily physical activity that is sustained over the course of the lifetime in human beings is evident. When activity energy expenditure is related to body size, levels of habitual physical activity fall with age in both males and females, beginning even

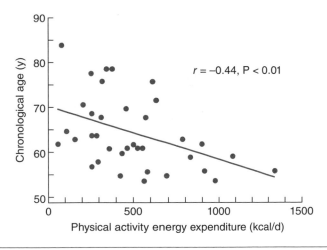

Figure 2.3   Daily physical activity energy expenditure measured by doubly labeled water plotted against chronological age in 44 older women.

Reprinted, by permission, from R.D. Starling, 2001, "Energy expenditure and aging: Effects of physical activity," *International Journal of Sport Nutrition and Exercise Metabolism* 11: S208-S217; data from Starling et al. 1998.

in the preschool years. The degree of decline is greatest in the early years of childhood and into adolescence. In the middle adult and older years, the curve of activity continues to fall but at a slower rate. In most studies, the rate of decline is greatest in males.

As noted previously, not all have concluded that such findings necessarily reflect biological control of habitual physical activity. Regarding athletic participation, Burton felt that "the dropping out of sport is a necessary part of the normal trial-and-error sampling procedure that youngsters employ in trying to find those activity or achievement domains they enjoy the most" (19, p. 246). Telama and Yang were in agreement:

> Although Burton's notion mainly concerned dropping out of organized sport, it can also be applied to physical activity in general. It is supported, among other things, by the results of time-budget studies indicating that whereas physical activity decreases with age, the time spent in other leisure time activities increases (141).

In interpreting the "physical activity patterns [which] become less satisfactory with increasing age" as reflecting modifiable individual choice in response to environmental, social, and psychological factors, this "erosion" of activity has been viewed by some as "extremely disappointing" (27, p. 1605).

The extent that this falling curve of activity with age in humans reflects inherent biological control versus extrinsic environmental influences could be tested by assessing physical activity across the life span in members of cultures that have been isolated from the technological advances of advanced societies. Estimates of activity energy expenditure have been published in such populations, but, unfortunately, age has not been considered as a variable (94).

PHYSICAL ACTIVITY OF ANIMALS

Insights into the nature and control of physical activity in humans have often been sought through observations of animal models (145). Variables influencing the components of energy balance, including activity energy expenditure, are more easily isolated for study in animals, thereby avoiding the multitude of confounding determinants that make human studies so challenging. Most of this research has been conducted with mice and rats. Information obviously impossible to gain in humans is facilitated—effects of pharmacological interventions and experimentally induced central nervous system lesions, for instance. Rodents, with their shorter life span, can also be selectively bred to assess genetic influences on activity. It has been assumed that evidence for genetic controllers of locomotor activity in these animals is transferable to humans, since evidence suggests that rodents and humans share about 75% of their genomes (88). Still, the extent that rodent findings can be safely extrapolated to human beings may not be unlimited (for example, motor activity in female rodents is greater than in males [145], while the converse is observed in humans).

Forms of Activity

It should be recognized that physical activity as analyzed in studies of animal behavior is not a straightforward construct. Locomotor behavior has been categorized by several means, particularly in caged rodents: wheel running, food-seeking behavior, exploratory behavior in new environments, and habituated spontaneous activity, for example. Although it might be assumed that each represents an expression of biological control, the research evidence suggests that such regulation might occur by different mechanisms. Different studies have used these various forms of activity as outcome markers, sometimes with disparate results. Similarly nonuniform are the techniques used for estimating animal activity. Several methods for quantifying activity have been employed, such as direct observation, telemetry, wheel rotation counts, and infrared beams.

In addition, it is not clear how different forms of animal activity might be considered parallel to human activity energy expenditure. Some have suggested that habituated spontaneous activity in animals might be equated to NEAT in humans. Wheel running in rodents, on the other hand, may be an expression of voluntary or addictive behavior, driven by reward incentives.

Such confounders notwithstanding, the collective animal data provide a broad support for the existence of brain centers that regulate involuntary motor activity. Still, the issues outlined previously have sometimes proven problematic for those attempting to create a coherent picture of the nature of biologic control of activity energy expenditure in human beings based on animal models.

Lifetime Activity

One of the strongest arguments that the descending curve of habitual energy expenditure through physical activity that occurs with age in humans is basically biological in nature is the observation that similar declines are observed throughout the animal kingdom. In fact, virtually all species in which this phenomenon has been studied demonstrate a reduction in motor activity through the life span. Animals, of course, lack voluntary (in the sense of planned and purposeful) activity. They do not reflect and then choose to take a walk instead of resting on the couch. No cognitive decision making goes into level of habitual activity. However, available data suggest that the *magnitude* of the fall in habitual physical activity with age parallels that of humans. Not only supporting a biologic control of activity, this observation provides a clue that a biological regulator of activity energy expenditure might act in humans largely through the control of extent of spontaneous activities or NEAT.

In 2000, Ingram provided a comprehensive review of the extant research literature on animal activity over the life span (64). In the animals most commonly studied, he concluded that an "age-related decline in laboratory rodent species is a well-established phenomenon" (p. 1623). In this review, he cited 23 published cross-sectional reports documenting an age-related fall in exploratory and home-cage (habitual) activity in rats and mice, studied by various techniques, including infrared sensors and motion detectors. The decrease in activity in both forms of exercise between 6 and 30 months of age was over 50%. Similar trends have been described in four longitudinal studies of home-cage activity in rodents.

Though rodents have been the most commonly studied animals, similar patterns have been found in a range of species. Bolanowski and colleagues described an age-related fall in activity of the nematode (*Caenorhabditis elegans*), a microscopic worm that lives underground with a mature lifetime of less than a month (13). To accomplish this, these investigators sat at a microscope and counted oscillations of the worm's body over the period of a minute serially over time. Waves per minute were found to fall dramatically and linearly with age.

Spontaneous activity declines with age in fruit flies (84) and house flies (161). Monkeys observed in a zoological park demonstrated marked diminution of both walking and jumping activity from age 2 to 24 years (66). The report by Head and others in a study of dog activity suggested that differences in lifetime patterns could be differentiated by breed (61). Exploratory behavior declined with age in pound-source mixed-breed dogs between 9 months and 10 years of age, but not in beagles. On the other hand, beagles, but not the mixed-breed dogs, demonstrated a decline in human interaction activity between the ages of 2 and 13 years.

Perhaps the only known exception to this pattern of decline of activity with age may be that of the giant squid. Little is known for certain regarding the behavior of these massive creatures, which live in deep water throughout the oceans, and are rarely observed. During an unusually short life span not exceeding about 5 years, they grow rapidly to a remarkable size (the largest on record is a body of 7.4 ft [2.3 m] with a total length, including tentacles, of 43 ft [13 m]). To achieve this, the growth rate of the squid is exponential throughout life, in distinction to the early maturation of most other members of the animal kingdom (5). This continual rapid growth can be expected to be paralleled by progressive increases in motor activity to obtain food to satisfy needs for caloric intake (oceanographer Grant Cumming, personal communication).

Further evidence that the decline in activity energy expenditure in animals represents a true biologically dictated phenomenon—governed by gene action—comes from the observation that mice selectively bred for physical activity may experience variations in the rate of decline in activity with age. Lhotellier and Cogen-Salmon showed that the pattern of diminished motor activity, measured by photocell beams, differed among three strains of mice bred for hyperactivity when evaluated at age 150 days (juvenile), 400 days (mature), and 750 days (senescent) (86).

Wheel Running

As noted previously, it is likely that the locomotor behavior of animals can be considered equivalent to spontaneous activities or NEAT in humans (57). However, wheel running by rodents, when such a device is placed in their cages, may serve as a special case. Specifically, just how this wheel running relates to the control of energy expenditure by spontaneous behavioral activities (defensive, aggressive, food seeking) and where such repetitious activity fits into the maintenance of energy balance (see part II) are uncertain. It has been noted that wheel running is rewarding to animals, that it can sometimes be related to rodent personality traits, and that it can be addictive (57). For this reason, wheel running has been proposed to represent a *stereotypic* behavior in that it is constant, repetitious, and lacking in any obvious goal (102). Some have contended, in fact, that "voluntary wheel running in rodents may be a reasonable model of human volitional exercise" (57, p. 207). Therefore, this activity might be instigated by factors such as exercise fitness and sensations of pain or pleasure. Novak and others contended that "wheel-running behavior represents factors in addition to rodents' tendency to be physically active, engaging additional neural and physiological mechanisms which can then independently alter energy balance and behavior" (107, p. 1001). How such stereotypic behavior and habitual spontaneous activities might be differentiated by biologic control is not understood.

Finally, Meijer and Robbers performed an interesting experiment in which a 24 cm diameter running wheel (along with camera, motion sensor, and food tray) was placed in an outdoor environment to determine if rodents would engage in wheel running in their natural environment (102). They found that, indeed, wild mice ran on the wheel, and with the same duration as mice in cages. Even more surprising perhaps was these authors' report that "wheel movement not caused by mice was caused by shrews, rats, snails, slugs, or frogs" (p. 2) that visited the testing site.

Rhodes and colleagues identified regions of the brain that define wheel-running behavior in mice (117). These authors compared immunoreactivity for FOS, which is expressed in response to neuronal stimulation, in the brains of mice selectively bred for voluntary wheel running to those of non-active control animals. Seven brain regions were considered as potentially responsible for the variation in wheel running between the two groups: the caudate-putamen complex, prefrontal cortex, medial frontal cortex, nucleus accumbens, piriform cortex, sensory cortex, and lateral hypothalamus. Other investigators have reported similar findings during treadmill running in rats (65, 90, 108).

Effects of Sex

A mong human beings, males have been observed to be more active than females in virtually every study that has examined sex influences on habitual physical activity. This finding has proven consistent independent of age, race, measurement technique, or definition of exercise intensity. For example, Sallis and colleagues found that boys were on the average 14% more active than girls in their review of nine studies assessing activity by self-report in youth 6 to 18 years old (126). When objective measures such as heart rate were utilized, the male predominance increased to 23%. In the four studies reviewed by Corder and Ekelund, which assessed activity by accelerometers in free-living conditions, activity in the youth 4 to 15 years old was greater in the males by 8% to 20% (31). The meta-analysis of 127 studies of physical activity in individuals between 2 months and 30 years of age by Eaton and Enns indicated significantly higher levels in males throughout, with the gap becoming greater with age (43). In this review, the average male was more active than 69% of the females.

This sex difference in level of physical activity has traditionally been attributed to the influence of sociocultural factors, particularly beginning in adolescence. At this time,

> Females face social pressures that have historically linked physical prowess and athleticism to maleness, and gender differences in activity have traditionally been accounted for by perceptions that femininity is not consistent with vigorous activity and sport play. In adolescence these influences are compounded by the burgeoning sexuality at puberty and strong desire for attractiveness to the opposite sex. In males, sexual desirability is often linked to physical capabilities in sports participation and physical activity. In females, on the other hand, attractiveness is focused on physical features, often perceived as incompatible with vigorous physical activity. (122, p. 3-4)

Two observations, however, suggest that such sex differences in physical activity might be at least partially biologically controlled—that there is something about one's numbers of X chromosomes that influences daily motor activity. First, evidence suggests that sex-related differences in activity might be at least partially explained by similar variations between males and females in rate of sexual maturation. This information supports the idea that biological effects—in this case, the effect of sex hormonal influences—contribute to sex differences in habitual physical activity beyond the influence of sociocultural factors. And, second, some information indicates that sex differences in motor activity might be evident within the first months of life and even *in utero*, well before any social influences could be expected to be effective.

SEXUAL MATURATION

The title of the 1989 publication by Eaton and Yu posed a provocative question: "Are sex differences in child motor activity level a function of sex differences in maturational status?" (44). By "maturational status," these authors were referring to level of biological maturation, defined as the progression of physical and functional traits toward the mature state (96). Included in this maturational process are a number of biological systems, including somatic growth (stature), osseous development (bone age), and sexual maturation (expressed directly as reproductive capacity and by secondary characteristics, such as breast and pubic hair development). For most individuals, full maturation in these different functions is achieved by the end of the teen years. The important points here are two: First, the age of onset and tempo or rate of biological maturation varies among individuals, and is not always consistent with chronological age. At the same age, then, youth may vary markedly in level of biological maturation—some are early maturers, others late maturers. Second, girls as a group reach markers of biological maturation at younger ages than boys, reaching peak height velocity and puberty 1 to 2 years in advance of their male classmates.

What Eaton and Yu were suggesting was that the lower activity levels traditionally observed in young females compared to males might be explained by the accelerated level of biological maturation in the former. To test this hypothesis, they examined the amount of habitual physical activity (by caretaker questionnaire) in respect to level of physical maturation (ratio of present height to estimated adult height) in 83 boys and girls aged 5 to 8 years. As expected, when plotted against chronological age, girls were less active yet more mature than the boys. When level of estimated biological maturation was considered, the sex effect on activity was reduced in magnitude but remained statistically significant. These authors concluded that "maturity is one of several mechanisms in the determination of sex differences in activity level" (44, p. 1010).

After this initial foray into the question, a number of studies have followed that have reinforced the concept that variation in biological maturation may help explain male–female differences in habitual motor activity during the growing years.

Using a mixed longitudinal design, Thompson and colleagues studied 70 boys and 68 girls over a 7-year span between ages 9 and 18 years (143). Physical activity was assessed by questionnaire and biological age by peak height velocity. By chronological age, boys were more active than girls. However, when adjusted for biological age, sex differences were eliminated, except at 3 years before peak height velocity. The authors concluded that this study "illuminates the influence of pubertal development on physical activity behaviors" (p. 1689).

Sherar and others sought to verify the role of biological maturation on sex differences in physical activity in a cross-sectional study of 194 boys and 207 girls aged 8 to 13 years (133). Physical activity level was directly measured by 7 days of accelerometer readings, and physical maturity was assessed by estimated peak height velocity (using an equation based on height, sitting height, and leg length). As expected, boys were more active than girls, and activity levels fell with age. However, when aligned with respect to level of physical maturation, sex differences in activity disappeared.

Similar results were obtained in the longitudinal study of Cairney and colleagues, who assessed 2,100 youth serially between the ages of 9 and 15 years (23). A questionnaire was used to determine time spent participating in physical activities (including free-time play, sport teams, and other organized activities). Biological maturation status was assessed by estimated age of peak height velocity. When findings were adjusted for maturation, the expected effects of age on activity levels by sex were eliminated. Other studies have consequently confirmed these findings (34).

The reports supported the concept that differences in level and rate of biological maturation contribute to sex differences (by chronological age) during the growing years. In this way, sex differences in physical activity during childhood and adolescence are explained by the differential tempo of sexual maturation in males and females, pointing to a biological rather than a sociocultural influence.

On the other hand, studies investigating the influence of biological maturation on levels of physical activity *within* each sex have produced conflicting results. In 2010, Sherar and others reviewed these reports, noting that at least six studies showed no influence of biological maturation on activity levels of adolescent girls, while others have reported an inverse relationship between the two (132). These authors suggested that these conflicting findings might reflect differences in variables such as activity measurement tool, nature of the study populations, small sample size, and subject psychosocial mediating factors.

Little data are available regarding the maturity–activity relationship in males. Such information might be expected to be confounded by the tendency for participation by early maturing boys in organized sports such as football and ice hockey, in which greater strength and speed offer a competitive advantage. In a longitudinal investigation, Cumming and colleagues found that advanced maturation (by percentage predicted adult height) in both males and females at age 11 years did not predict physical activity levels (by accelerometer counts) at age 13 years (33).

No clear explanation has been found for any connection that might exist between level of biologic maturation and habitual physical activity. Indeed, Cumming has contended that "a criticism of research examining relations between biological maturation and physical activity in youth is that it is largely atheoretical, lacking a clear conceptual framework from which to explain and interpret findings" (32, p. 130).

The simplest explanation for the sex difference in activity levels at a given age in young people would be this: If the expected fall in habitual activity over time is related to level of biological development, females, being advanced by 2 years compared to males of the same chronological age, would simply be farther along the declining trajectory. This would not, however, explain the inconsistency of findings in intragender studies examining the influence of maturation status and activity levels. Nor would such an explanation serve to explain sex differences in activity that persist in life after the age of maturity has been attained.

To seek an etiologic basis of sex differences in activity in the hormonal responses at puberty with the activation of the hypothalamic–pituitary–gonadal axis is intuitively tempting. However, as reviewed by Bowen and others (16), the data in humans are sparse and inconclusive. In humans, estrogen levels can influence mood and pain threshold, but estrogenic influence on physical activity levels—increased or decreased—has not been clearly established (16, 118). Similarly, studies examining the influence of testosterone on habitual motor activity in humans are lacking.

Studies in animals indicate that females are more active than males as a result of hormonal (estrogen) effects. In animals, estrogen administration is recognized to *increase* rather than diminish levels of motor activity, and this observation has been used to explain the higher levels of activity in female animals compared to males (87). However, it all might not be that simple, since testosterone also serves to enhance physical activity in animals (58). It may be, for instance, that administered testosterone is metabolically converted to estrogen, thereby stimulating activity (125). Such findings clearly indicate the biological basis of sex differences in motor activity in animals. In humans, the reverse is observed—males are more active than females throughout the life span, even among small infants. Whether there is a hormonal explanation for this pattern has not been adequately studied.

It is possible that secondary effects of augmented estrogen levels at puberty could diminish activity levels in humans, such as greater accumulation of body fat. Cumming suggested, too, that psychosocial influences linked to biological maturation that become prominent in adolescence may have an effect on desire to participate in physical activities, such as self-concept, body image, and peer acceptance (32).

Obviously, future investigations to define hormonal pathways that define sex differences in humans are needed. As Bowen and colleagues concluded,

> The clinical implications of expanding this research are potentially far reaching. Currently a large body of literature exists regarding how extrinsic and environmental factors influence physical activity levels in humans. Unfortunately beneficial alterations to health indicators are minimal, and physical inactivity and related conditions remain disproportionately high. Thus, physical management strategies and research agenda that focus solely on environmental or extrinsic factors remain shortsighted. The overall goal of physical activity-sex hormone interaction research should be to further delineate biological pathways and identify enzymes/proteins/biomolecules involved in up-regulating activity levels in humans. (16, p. 9)

SEX DIFFERENCES IN INFANCY

That greater average levels of activity are observed in human males than females from very early on in infancy—assumedly preceding the opportunity for any significant sociocultural influences—has been considered evidence of a biological influence on daily activity energy expenditure (24). Individual studies examining this issue have generally lacked sufficient number of subjects and often utilized questionable parent report, prompting the performance of two meta-analyses. The first, published in 1986, was composed of 14 studies (43). This revealed a mean effect size (an indicator of biological significance) indicating a greater activity level in males in studies of infants between 0 and 11 months of age of 0.29, which differed significantly from zero ($p < 0.001$). The second, by Campbell and Eaton in 1999, was performed to increase the number of studies assessed as well as examine the influences of age and measurement technique (24). This review included 46 studies from 1984 to 1998, which comprised 78 sex difference comparisons (not all independent) of infants during the first year of life. Consistent with the earlier meta-analysis, the average male infant was found to be more active than the average female (effect size for 78 comparisons was 0.12, with 95% confidence limits significantly greater than zero). Although sex differences were significant, a considerable overlap was evident in male and female activity. The median male exhibited greater level of activity than 58% of the females.

No significant differences between the two sexes were evident by modality of measurement in the meta-analysis, but the effect size for subjective parent ratings (0.09) was less than half of that seen by using observational measures (0.20) or objectively by instrumentation (0.21). The magnitude of the sex difference remained stable throughout the first year of life. The authors concluded,

> Given such convergent data, we favour the interpretation that these early sex differences are largely innate and biological in origin. . . . This early sex difference presumably influences, and interacts with, gender-specific socialization processes to amplify sex differences as the child ages. (24, p. 12)

The conclusion that early sex differences in motor activity have a biological basis would be supported if similar findings could be identified prior to birth (i.e., differential levels of fetal activity). On this point, the published data have not provided a consistent picture. In the 1986 meta-analysis of sex differences in motor activity in prenatal studies by Eaton and Enns, males were more active, but the mean effect size was 0.33, which did not differ significantly from zero (43). However, this included only six studies, which was felt to be inadequate for answering the question.

Almli and others found that males were more active than females when they made longitudinal observations of fetal leg movements per minute by ultrasonography at 30, 34, and 37 weeks gestation (3). Robles de Medina and colleagues performed ultrasound measurements of 56 male and 67 female fetuses for general movements over 1 hour at 15 to 17 and 27 to 28 weeks gestation and for 2 hours at 37 to 39 weeks gestation (120). No significant differences were observed between males and females except for a higher percent time in movement in the males at term. However, the latter finding lost statistical significance after correcting for time of fetal wakefulness, which was greater in the males.

Neurochemical Models

An extensive volume of research has focused on identifying the neurochemical pathways that influence habitual physical activity in both animals and humans. Understandably, most of these investigations have involved animals; many have examined patterns of change over time in such mechanisms that might be linked to declines of activity over the life span. These data clearly support the existence of biologic control. Still, one awaits a comprehensive picture of just how this biologic controller might work. This chapter outlines a number of the best-supported possible mechanisms. The identification of the mechanistic basis of a central governor that operates to regulate activity energy expenditure is further addressed in chapter 10.

DOPAMINE

Much research attention has been centered on the actions of dopamine-dependent neural mechanisms in the brain that alter regular motor activity. Dopamine is a catecholamine related (and metabolized) to norepinephrine and epinephrine. In the brain it serves as a *neurotransmitter*, a chemical agent that connects signals from one nerve cell (neuron) to the next across a synapse. There dopamine is responsible for multiple excitatory functions, including the rush from a morning coffee, the euphoria of falling in love, and the cravings of narcotic addiction.

The extent of actions of dopamine is contingent on both the level of its secretion by nerve endings and the density of dopamine receptors (labeled as D1-D5) on receiving neurons. Most attention, in fact, has focused on alterations of dopamine receptor function in its association with variations in motor activity. The level of action of dopamine receptors has been linked to administration of pharmacologic agents, amount of dopamine in the system, sexual activity, and—of particular interest to exercise scientists—

motor activity and its limits. Foley and colleagues demonstrated elevated dopamine-related receptor mRNA in rats that had been bred for a superior level of endurance performance capacity, raising implications for the role of central factors in defining exercise fatigue (53).

Dopamine-secreting neurons are clustered in various locations in the brain, each with its own particular actions. Regarding control of spontaneous physical activity, interest has centered on two: the pars compacta of the substantia nigra, a small area in the basal ganglia, which appears to regulate habitual motor activity, and the ventral tegmental area (VTA) in the midbrain, which controls levels of motivation and reward-seeking motor behavior. Thus, dopamine-secreting neurons in the brain could conceptually alter physical activity levels either or both by (a) directly stimulating efferent motor pathways and (b) creating motivation for exercise by reinforcing physical behavior through reward (pleasure) (figure 4.1).

Each of these two centers extends its influence to multiple brain target areas. As Knab and Lightfoot have described,

From an anatomical perspective, it is important to point out that locomotor control areas of the brain (striatum, nigro-striatal pathways) and reward/motivational areas of the brain (nucleus accumbens,

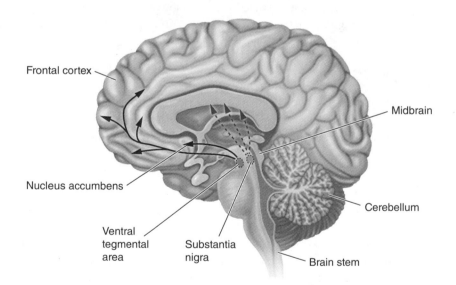

Figure 4.1 Anatomic location of dopamine centers in the brain in the nigrostriatal tract (considered to control motor movement) and the ventral tegmental area (VTA) felt to be involved in physical activity in response to motivation and reward. Neuronal tracts disseminate widely from these centers to other areas of the brain.

ventral tegmental area) are integrated by neural connections through regions such as the ventral pallidum. Thus, although collectively the basal ganglia neurons control distinct areas of the brain, these regions do not act in isolation, and it is certainly likely that motivation for exercise involves an integrated control from several of these regions. (76, p. 142)

Animal Studies

Dopamine is detected in a number of unicellular organisms and has been found to modify motor behavior throughout the animal kingdom. For this reason, it has been assumed that dopamine-related systems in the brain as determinants of locomotion have a very long evolutionary history (7).

In examining animal studies relating dopamine systems to locomotor behavior, it is useful to remember the issues described in chapter 2 regarding the vagaries of measurement techniques and types of motor activity in nonhuman species, particularly rodents, and the uncertainty of how these relate to specific categories of nonvolitional activities in humans. As Garland and others noted,

> Various neural correlates of generalized locomotor activity have long been the subject of considerable research, but central themes are difficult to extract, often because operational definitions of locomotor activity vary widely. . . . One needs to be extremely careful when reading the literature to note what a particular study actually means by "locomotor activity," as it is often used to describe either activity in home cages after a period of acclimation or habituation, locomotion in acute tests in novel arenas (e.g., open-field tests), or even wheel running. (57, pp. 208, 213)

Pertinent to the present discussion, it is possible that different neurochemical mechanisms might underlie these different forms of motor activities.

Several lines of inquiry have examined the role of dopamine in the control of locomotor activity in animals:

• Volume of wheel running in genetically active rodents is linked to an augmented dopaminergic effect. For instance, Bronikowski and colleagues reported a 20% increase in dopamine receptors D2 and D4 in mice selected for high levels of wheel running compared to control mice (17). Fink and Reis described higher levels of dopamine activity in the nigrostriatal and mesolimbic pathways in the brains of mice with greater wheel-running activity (52). Differences in expression of D1 receptors that separated active from inactive animals have been described by Knab and others (75). Waters and colleagues found that selectively bred, highly fit rats that exhibited greater wheel running had greater dopamine activity in the striatum area of the brain (153).

• In studies of rats, electrical stimulation of the substantia nigra and ventral tegmental area triggers increases in spontaneous activity (81).

• Administration of dopamine antagonists, either systemically or into the nucleus accumbens, has been described by several authors to diminish open-field and spontaneous activity in rats (57).

• Parallel declines in motor activity and dopamine system function are observed as animals (and humans) age. Roth and Joseph have reviewed data indicating that this fall in dopamine neuronal activity is predominantly an outcome of decreased densities of dopamine receptors (121). Decline in number of dopamine-secreting neurons is also involved. In one study, receptor and neuronal losses were 35% and 20%, respectively, in rats ages 6 months to 24 months. This information provides a possible neurochemical basis for the ubiquitous fall in energy expenditure through physical activity during the animal life span.

Although the association of motor activity and action of dopamine systems in the brain in animals seems incontrovertible, two important questions surrounding research efforts need to be considered. First, are the actions of dopamine a direct cause or a secondary response to physical activity? Second, how much of dopamine's action serves instead to motivate activity through reward and reinforcement? These issues arise when considering dopamine mechanisms for stimulating physical activity in humans.

Human Studies

In the title of their 2010 article, Knab and Lightfoot posed this question: "Does the difference between physically active and couch potato lie in the dopamine system?" (76). More to the point, is the evidence indicating a central role of dopamine systems in controlling the physical activity of animals transferable to human beings?

Experimental evidence to this point is, as might be expected, very limited. It is generally accepted that the dopamine system is activated by physical activity. In their review, Knab and Lightfoot concluded,

It is clear that the dopaminergic system is affected by physical activity, and [while] it is plausible that the amount of voluntary physical activity is regulated at least in part by the dopamine system . . . evidence is still lacking as to whether the dopamine system is actually working in an independent role in influencing voluntary physical activity (e.g., can dopaminergic difference *cause* changes in motivated physical activity in humans). (76, pp. 142-43)

Similar conclusions hold for involuntary or spontaneous activity.

Nonetheless, some observations support the idea that dopamine activity in the brain acts in a direct manner to control levels of physical activity levels in humans, which has been documented in animals. Parallel declines in habitual physical activity and function of the dopamine system, explained by a decrease in dopamine receptor activity, are observed as humans age (121). Patients with Parkinson's disease suffer from motor impairment and diminished activity, caused by loss of dopamine-secreting neurons in the substantia nigra. Clinical improvement is often observed in Parkinson's patients after treatment with the chemical L-DOPA, which is converted to dopamine in the brain. Motor disorders such as attention deficit hyperactivity disorder (ADHD), restless legs syndrome, and anorexia nervosa have been linked to abnormalities of dopamine function (see chapter 5 for discussion).

There is reason to expect that the reward and reinforcement actions of dopamine are operant in humans as well. Regular exercise is a well-documented way to alleviate symptoms of depression. Runners describe feelings of euphoria after their workouts and competitions (the runner's high). For some people, regular exercise can be addictive, and in the absence of regular physical activity, these people experience withdrawal symptoms.

However, Huppertz and others could find no association between gene alleles affecting dopamine receptors and leisure-time exercise behavior in a study of 8,768 individuals in the Netherlands Twin Register Study (62). This report was limited to time spent in voluntary, self-initiated physical activities assessed by questionnaire instead of general physical activity levels. From this perspective, this study failed to support a role for the dopaminergic reward system in motivating such activities.

OTHER NEUROCHEMICAL MEDIATORS

Many other neurochemical mediators that appear to influence levels of motor activity have been identified, mainly in animal models. In 2008, Teske and colleagues (142) compiled a list of 26 such agents, the number of which has presumably risen during the process of publication of this book. As Garland and others stated, "Various correlates of generalized locomotor activity have long been the subject of considerable research, but central themes are difficult to extract" (57, p. 213). Moreover, most of these proposed mediators have been identified in studies related to energy balance, particularly weight change and appetite, and not specifically to activity energy expenditure through motor activity. In sum, researchers are not at a loss for candidate agents for participation in the control of motor activity, but what each of these agents might mean in the regulation of activity energy expenditure is not at all clear. The following are brief descriptions of several mediators most likely to play key roles in physical activity behavior.

Orexin-A

Orexin-A is a peptide that is synthesized in the lateral hypothalamus, with widespread projections throughout the brain (57, 80). Spontaneous activity of mice is augmented when orexin is injected into specific brain areas, and motor activity in animals lacking orexin is reduced (142). Orexin gene–deleted mice demonstrate reduced levels of spontaneous activity. To truly challenge the skeptical, an overexpression of orexin stimulates increased motor activity in zebrafish (115). Kotz and colleagues declared, in fact, that "the most well-established NEAT generator to date is hypothalamic orexin A" (80, p. R701). Orexin-A does communicate with the substantia nigra and paraventricular nuclei, so it is possible that dopamine secretion might serve as a final outcome agent for the role of orexin-A in promoting motor activity. Supporting this, physical activity in animals stimulated by orexin-A is abolished by the dopamine receptor blockade (81).

Melanocortin Receptors

The influence of the melanocortin system in controlling energy balance is indicated by reports of alteration in activity in both humans and animals when this system is disturbed (20, 47). Melanocortin receptors are linked with several neuropeptides (including leptin and neuropeptide Y) in the hypothalamus and other brain regions to particularly influence caloric intake and weight gain in animals. Hwa and colleagues demonstrated that infusion of a melanocyte receptor agonist in lean Zucker rats raised 3-hour total activity counts by 50% and 3-hour oxygen content (expressed relative to kg body mass$^{0.75}$) by 30% (63).

Ghrelin

Ghrelin is a peptide synthesized in the stomach that may act to modulate physical activity through its actions on hypothalamic centers in the brain. Its effects on activity have not been fully clarified. Ghrelin-deficient mice have been described to exhibit no change in activity levels, but injections of this peptide into the brain have provoked a reduction in locomotor activity. Other reports describe acute stimulatory effects on motor activity. Kotz and others suggested that the discrepancies between these studies might relate to the duration of activity measurement after ghrelin injection (80).

Nitric Oxide

Some data indicate that nitric oxide plays a role in modulating motor behavior. Systemic injections of inhibitors of nitric oxide synthase, the enzyme that promotes nitric oxide formation, have been demonstrated to decrease rat maze exploration as well as motor activity in open-field studies. It has been suggested that nitric oxide may modulate motor activity by its influence on dopaminergic neuronal activity in the substantia nigra (39).

Thorburn and Proietto noted that actions of estrogen and nitric oxide covary—that is, a fall in estrogen levels reduces nitric oxide production in animals, while estrogen replacement restores nitric oxide concentrations (144). They suggested that a fall in motor activity caused by reduced estrogen in animals might be mediated by depleted nitric oxide.

Other Polypeptides and Pharmacologic Agents

Stimulant effects on spontaneous physical activity of rodents have been ascribed to a variety of other polypeptides that can influence neural transmission in the brain. These include cholecystokinin, corticotropin-releasing hormone, neuromedin U, neuropeptide Y, and agouti-related protein (142). Leptin, which may play a role in appetite and body composition, appears to help regulate motor behavior in animals but not in humans. For example, administered leptin augments physical activity in leptin-deficient mice, but similar effects are not observed in humans with low levels of leptin (67, 144). Viggiano has commented that "apparently the alteration of any neurotransmitter system can increase locomotor activity" (149, p. 4).

Certain deficiency and toxic states have been associated with alterations in habitual physical activity. Rats with iron deficiency exhibit alterations in their light–dark circadian activity patterns, an observation that Beard considered "of great interest because it implies a perturbance of a basic hypothalamic control process" (9, p. 73). This finding might reflect the iron dependence of the synthetic metabolic pathways of brain neurotransmitters or their receptors. In addition, lead poisoning in both animals and humans has been associated with increased motor activity. Silbergeld and Goldberg reported that suckling mice that were fed lead acetate demonstrated activity levels that were three times that of control animals (134).

Viggiano (149), as well as Thorburn and Proietto (144), outlined an extensive list of pharmacologic agents and biochemical agents whose actions have been associated with hyperactive and hypoactive behavior in both animals and humans. Those biological agents that can modulate levels of habitual motor activity in humans and animals include the following [from Thorburn and Proietto (144), Viggiano (149)]:

Agents Causing Hyperactivity	Agents Causing Hypoactivity
• Pancreatic polypeptide	• Estrogen insufficiency
• Melatonin	• Deficient histamine receptors
• Acetyl-L-carnitine	• Low-dose noradrenaline
• D-glucosamine	• Serotonin (short-term)
• High-dose noradrenaline	• Fibroblast growth factor
• Serotonin (long-term)	• Brain-derived neurotrophic factor
• Nerve growth factor	• Adenosine
• Pentobarbital	• Opioid receptor blockade
• Diazepam	• Acetylcholine
• Thyroid hormone	• Hypothyroidism
• Corticosterone	
• Hyperuricemia	

These observations of chemical effects on activity support the existence of a biologic controller. However, as Panksepp and colleagues cautioned, alterations in motor activity from such agents might be simply a manifestation of changes in synaptic activity that are "pushed outside the range of normal transmission patterns" (110, p. 473).

Viggiano noted that given such a pervasive effect on activity levels by so many agents, it was challenging to provide a unitary view of how all might influence motor behavior (149). In the end, he suggested, they each might act by means of a different mechanism.

Certainly the information provided in this chapter cannot be tied up neatly in a single conceptual package, and a great number of gaps exist in the understanding of neurochemical mechanisms for controlling activity expenditure. Still, taken collectively, these data provide strong evidence for the existence of such biological control. As Teske and others concluded, "Studies in both animals and humans suggest that the level of spontaneous physical activity and NEAT is innate and under the biological regulation [of] several brain nuclei and their associated neuromodulators and neurotransmitters" (142, p. 84).

Perturbations of Brain Function

C ertain derangements of brain function—both experimentally induced and naturally occurring—have been demonstrated to affect levels of activity energy expenditure. This chapter describes alterations in activity level observed following focal lesions in the brains of animals, hypothalamic tumors, and disturbances of regulation of habitual motor activity in patients with anorexia nervosa, restless legs syndrome, and attention deficit hyperactivity disorder (ADHD). In each situation, a case can be made for perturbation of a biologic regulator of habitual activity, both in animals and humans, that alters activity energy expenditure.

LESIONS IN ANIMAL BRAINS

Alterations of levels of habitual motor activity have been described after the creation of experimentally induced lesions in the brains of animals (110, 149). Viggiano listed studies indicating lesions in 12 brain regions that resulted in stimulated motor activity but found fewer that diminished activity levels (149). Extensive lesions in the amygdala have predictably lowered spontaneous motor activity in rats. Septal lesions, on the other hand, result in animal hyperactivity. A decline in play activity has been reported after damage to the dorsomedial thalamus, parafascicular area of the thalamus, and caudate nucleus. After hypophysectomy, exploratory behavior increases in rats. Rodents become markedly hypoactive after removal of the caudate nucleus.

Particular interest has focused on alterations of motor activity in animals after experimental injury to the hypothalamus, since this region is recognized to control energy intake and play a central role in energy balance. Studies assessing outcomes of electrolytic injury, radio frequency lesions, and surgical incision of the ventromedial hypothalamus in rodents have been reviewed by Tou and Wade (145). Following such lesions, animals become hyperphagic and develop significant obesity. Concomitantly, levels of physical activity decline. It is not clear whether this decrease in activity reflects a compensatory control mechanism for disturbed appetite (i.e., increases in energy in) or a direct effect of hypothalamic injury, or whether it is simply an effect of excess body weight. It should be noted that some investigations have revealed that obesity may develop in such lesioned animals without evidence of high energy intake. This suggests that depressed levels of motor activity in such animals might represent a primary rather than a secondary effect.

Concussions may also affect activity levels in animals. Budinich and colleagues found an effect of traumatic brain injury on motor activity of male mice (18). After a controlled cortical impact, the animals were observed to become hyperactive in an open-field situation.

The diversity of disturbed loci that can alter activity energy expenditure in animals, much like the long list of chemical agents producing similar effects noted in chapter 4, speaks to the complexity of mechanisms within the central nervous system that can influence levels of habitual physical activity. Panksepp and others have pointed out that these outcomes might reflect global behavioral changes rather than disturbances of specific brain systems responsible for motor behavior (110).

CRANIOPHARYNGIOMA

Understandably, information regarding physical activity outcomes following experimentally induced lesions in the central nervous system is not available in human beings. Even in those with intracranial pathology (such as space-occupying masses or cerebral vascular accidents), any reports of alterations in habitual activity would likely be confounded by factors such as medications and their side effects, associated abnormalities (such as anemia), psychological disturbances, influence of pathology on motor capacity, and sleep disturbances. For example, acromegaly is a condition in humans reflecting increased secretion of growth factors, typically from a somatotropic pituitary tumor. Patients with acromegaly typically exhibit depression of regular physical activity, but in the study of 42 adult patients by Dantas and colleagues, joint pain inhibiting motor activities was reported in more than 80% of patients (35). And in the report of Orsey and colleagues of 36 children aged 8 to 18 years with cancer (23 with leukemia or lymphoma, 5 with brain tumors, 8 with solid tumors), physical activity levels were inversely related to quality of sleep (109).

Still, there is one story of brain tumor effect on level of habitual physical activity in humans that may prove instructive. Craniopharyngioma is a tumor in the region of the pituitary and hypothalamus at the base of the brain that affects the young (5 to 14 years of age) and the elderly (50 to 74 years of age). Approximately half of patients who undergo extirpation of the tumors develop obesity, and hyperphagia has traditionally been considered the explanation for this reflection of energy imbalance. This situation, then, is analogous to the experimental hypothalamic lesions described previously in animals.

Harz and colleagues attempted to decipher the mechanisms underlying obesity in 19 young patients who had undergone treatment for craniopharyngioma matched for age and body mass index with healthy control subjects (59). Daily physical activity was assessed by accelerometer, and a validated 1-week food diary was completed to estimate caloric intake. Average daily energy intake was 1,916 to 2,075 kcal in the craniopharyngioma patients and 2,476 in the controls. The former demonstrated fewer movement counts than the latter in the clinical setting (mean 228 vs. 298 counts/min) and in the outpatient setting (228 vs. 282 counts/min).

The findings indicated, in contrast to expectations, that reduced physical activity rather than greater caloric intake was responsible for the obesity associated with craniopharyngioma in this group of patients. In their discussion of these results, the authors postulated several possible mechanisms for this reduction in activity energy expenditure, including damage to hypothalamic control centers, low thyroid hormone, associated neurological and visual defects, and alterations in autonomic activity.

ANOREXIA NERVOSA

Patients with anorexia nervosa are characterized by compulsive resistance to eating or binge eating and purging behaviors. In addition, hyperactivity is commonly observed with this disorder, evident in up to 80% of cases (82). This condition thus represents an interesting paradox, since an inherent drive for body energy balance would be expected to trigger a compensatory decline in habitual motor activity as caloric intake falls. The increased physical activity engaged in by those with anorexia nervosa has often been considered as part of a purposeful strategy to lose weight; that is, the same compulsive need to refuse to eat dictates an addictive requirement to exercise. Several studies, in fact, have linked obsessive beliefs about eating with obsessive beliefs about exercise in these patients (38, 104).

Others have suggested that this hyperactivity is biologic in origin, most specifically an expression of disturbed dopamine function (26, 37). This argument is supported by findings of excessive motor activity in animal models of anorexia nervosa. For example, in the activity-based anorexia model, food restriction of rats and mice stimulates increased wheel running, which results in significant weight loss as a consequence of the combined effects of caloric restriction and excess motor activity (1). In these animals, the level of increased motor activity has been directly associated with the extent of food restriction. In various reports, such mice have been found to demonstrate low levels of leptin, reduction of thyroid hormone, increased hypothalamic serotonin secretion, and high levels of hydrocortisone (77). It has been suggested that the augmented motor behavior in these animals as well as humans in the face of caloric deprivation represents a primitive response of a drive to increase food-searching behavior (26).

Another anorexia mouse model (anx/anx) is a mutant that displays both diminished appetite and hyperactivity. Investigations in these animals have demonstrated several central nervous system changes, including alterations in dopaminergic, serotonergic, and noradrenergic systems, as well as neuro-degenerative changes in the hypothalamus. Other mouse anorexia mutants, including those with induced dopamine deficiency, are characterized by hypoactivity.

Considering the serious health effects of anorexia nervosa, considerable research efforts in humans have been directed toward understanding its underlying causal mechanisms with the goal of identifying effective thera-peutic modalities. Kontis and Theochari have reviewed current research investigations of neuroendocrine factors that might be responsible for the eating disorder and hyperactivity in patients with anorexia nervosa (78). Taken collectively, this information is confusing, with conflicting results and no clear common etiologic mechanism identified. The role of disturbed dopamine system function has long been suspected (8). Plasma concentra-tions of dopamine have been noted to rise during an exacerbation of anorexia nervosa, but urinary concentrations are reportedly normal or decreased. Positron emission tomography scanning has revealed higher dopamine receptor binding in the anteroventral striatum in women who have recovered from anorexia nervosa compared to healthy controls.

At present, then, there is evidence of disturbed central nervous system biological factors in both humans and animal models of anorexia nervosa with hyperactivity. However, no clear-cut neurochemical mechanism has been described. Consequently, as summarized by Kontis and Theochari in their review of 49 published studies, no consistently effective pharmacologic intervention has yet been identified (78). In particular, no therapeutic success has been observed after administration of dopamine agonists to patients with anorexia nervosa.

RESTLESS LEGS SYNDROME

Individuals with restless legs syndrome (RLS) have intense restlessness, paresthesias, and unpleasant creeping sensations in the lower extremities. These symptoms are usually nocturnal, compelling patients to rise from their beds and walk about (46). RLS is often familial, and several gene loci have been identified that are associated with this disorder.

The cause of RLS remains uncertain. However, pieces of evidence have been presented that have incriminated a disorder of dopamine function in the brain as responsible for this disorder (see ref. 36 for review). For example, Connor and colleagues examined the substantia nigra and putamen from autopsies of eight elderly patients with RLS whose onset of symptoms ranged from age 4 to 44 years (29). There they found a reduction of dopamine receptors that was directly related to the severity of RLS symptoms, as well as high levels of tyrosine hydroxylase, the enzyme responsible for synthesis of dopamine from tyrosine in the brain. Dopaminergic drugs have been helpful in reducing symptoms in some patients.

The other consistent finding in RLS, both in humans and animal models, has been a significant reduction in intracerebral iron content. There exists, in fact, a considerable amount of research evidence linking function of dopamine systems with brain iron status. Connor and colleagues showed that iron-deficient rats had higher levels of tyrosine hydroxylase than normally fed controls, a finding identical to cells in culture after iron chelation (29). These authors concluded that "the results are consistent with the hypothesis that a primary iron deficiency produces a dopaminergic abnormality characterized as an overly activated dopaminergic system as part of the RLS pathology" (p. 2403).

ATTENTION DEFICIT HYPERACTIVITY DISORDER

ADHD is another condition characterized by excessive motor activity—along with poor impulse control and learning problems—that is considered to be an expression of disturbed dopamine and catecholamine function in the central nervous system. Although it was initially assumed that those with ADHD suffered from excessive levels of brain arousal, it was subsequently recognized that central nervous stimulants such as amphetamine and methylphenidate acted to *relieve* signs of hyperactivity. This seemingly paradoxical observation provided a clue that the genesis of ADHD was more complicated than originally assumed.

More than 40 years ago, Satterfield and colleagues suggested that patients with ADHD suffered, in fact, from a state of *depressed* arousal (130). Along with others (60), they hypothesized that such low arousal reflected a defect in function of the reticular activating system, which triggered a rise in level of physical activity as stimulus-seeking strategy.

Since that time, a great deal of research has addressed the causal mechanisms underlying ADHD. Despite this, as Kieling and colleagues have noted, "Notwithstanding the empiric research on the identification of etiologic factors and the achievement of some remarkable well-replicated findings, comprehensive testable theories remain underspecified" (73, p. 286). Nonetheless, certain observations have proven important:

• ADHD appears to have a strong genetic basis. Twin studies have indicated heritability estimates of approximately 0.80. Most, however, consider ADHD as an outcome of complex genetic–environmental interactions; that is, "the genetic effect may only become apparent among the subgroup of individuals exposed to a certain environmental risk" (73, p. 290).

• Anatomically, brain imaging studies have indicated structural and functional abnormalities in the prefrontal cortex–basal ganglia–cerebellum circuit. In several neuroimaging studies, these structures have been found to demonstrate reduced metabolic rate and smaller size in patients with ADHD than in healthy individuals.

• A catecholamine imbalance is fundamental to most theories of ADHD causality (114). This is derived from several lines of evidence (see refs. 73, 159 for reviews). Several genes associated with ADHD have been identified, and these are recognized to control dopamine receptor function, the action of dopamine beta-hydroxylase (which converts dopamine to norepinephrine), and the dopamine transporter. The role of the latter has attracted particular research interest (92). The dopamine active transporter (DAT) gene controls uptake of dopamine at the synapse after its release from nerve endings, and mice lacking DAT demonstrate increased dopamine function. Some studies have shown elevated levels of DAT in the brain stratum of patients with ADHD. Stimulants such as amphetamine and methylphenidate, which are effective agents in reducing hyperactivity in patients with ADHD, block DAT and increase levels of dopamine at the synapse.

• Others have viewed ADHD as an outcome of abnormal connectivity. Imaging studies have suggested that ADHD is associated with abnormalities in white matter (the wiring portion of the brain) as well as with disruption of interactions of frontostriatal and mesocorticolimbic networks that could give rise to symptoms of ADHD (91).

Butte and colleagues documented that pharmacologic treatment in patients with ADHD actually reduced daily activity energy expenditure (21). They assessed total energy expenditure in a room calorimeter and physical activity by microwave motion detectors in 31 children with ADHD aged 6 to 12 years, both with and without stimulant medication treatment. Activities in the chamber consisted of riding a stationary bicycle, watching movies, and doing homework. Total energy expenditure decreased by 4% to 8% and physical activity decreased by 16% to 22% while taking medications.

The pathophysiology of ADHD remains incompletely delineated. However, this condition provides another example of derangement of brain neurochemical mechanisms that results in altered levels of habitual motor activity (150). Such models of normal function gone awry in the guise of human disease provide good evidence for biologic regulation of activity energy expenditure in the healthy central nervous system.

Organized Variability

egular rhythmic variability of physiologic function over time is an essential feature of all living beings. The most obvious of these intrinsic automatic patterns are *circadian rhythms*, the cyclic rise and fall of function over a day's time. If a person is isolated in a cave deprived of all effects of the light cycles of night and day, physiological rhythms occur in cycles of about 24 hours and 15 minutes. In the real world outside of the cave, however, this intrinsic periodicity is entrained by extrinsic stimuli—particularly light–dark cycles, sleeping, and eating—to a more precise 24-hour duration.

Other rhythmic temporal variations are often evident as well, such as recurring sequential patterns over shorter time spans. Seasonal hibernation is an example of regular variability on a longer-term basis (137). Although the explanation for such changes is often obscure, such organized variation in function is a central feature of both the plant and animal kingdoms, and its absence is associated with biologic dysfunction (154). If a biologic controller of physical activity exists, one would expect, then, to observe regular temporal patterns within the variability of motor activity.

ANIMAL CIRCADIAN RHYTHMS

Circadian rhythms are ubiquitous in both plants and animals. These diurnal patterns are evident even in individual cells, each of which has its own clock that controls phasic alterations in cell function. Underpinning each of these functions is a complex genetic mechanism (139). It has been noted that a majority of the 49 recognized hormone receptors in cells exhibits circadian rhythmicity (116). While influencing certain local functions, these individual clocks are coordinated and superseded by a master clock in the suprachiasmatic nucleus in the brain.

Circadian rhythms in physical activity have been documented widely throughout the animal kingdom. The list includes fiddler crabs, flying squirrels, fruit flies, iguanas, scorpions, rats, crayfish, spiny eels, hamsters, unicellular cyanobacteria, goldfish, and bees (42). Single-gene mutations have been identified that underlie these rhythms. For instance, the tau mutation in a hamster will change its periodicity of running from 24 hours to 20 hours. Experimental evidence indicates that these activity circadian rhythms are intrinsic but are modified by extrinsic factors. As early as 1939, Johnson reported that a mouse placed in continuous darkness will continue to demonstrate a periodicity of spontaneous activity, thereby "shown not to be dependent on any recognized or uncontrolled daily variable in the environment" (68, p. 321).

A number of observations in animals have revealed the influence of neurochemical mediators on this periodicity of motor behavior. The expression of orexin-A influences circadian rhythms in fish (106). Dopamine depletion results in disturbed or even abolished circadian rhythms (51). There is evidence in mice that ghrelin receptors may modulate circadian rhythms for free-running behavior (83). Biochemical mediators have been identified that cause light entrainment in the circadian rhythms of the cockroach (131).

In animals, then, locomotor behavior clearly exhibits circadian rhythmicity. But the converse also appears to be true—like light–dark cycles, physical activity can serve to entrain, or synchronize, circadian periodicity. Placing a rodent on a regular regimen of treadmill or wheel running has been reported to alter entrained activity rhythms of those animals kept under constant darkness (156).

HUMAN CIRCADIAN RHYTHMS

In humans, documenting circadian periodicity of daily activity energy expenditure is difficult, given the large number of influencing variables such as sleep and eating patterns, occupation, and scheduled physical activities. As part of the Baltimore Longitudinal Study on Aging, Xiao and colleagues measured daily patterns of physical activity of 773 free-living adults aged 31 to 96 years (157). Activity was assessed by accelerometry, with recordings in 1-minute epochs over 7 days. Consistent with sleep–awake cycles, a biphasic pattern of activity was observed, with a nadir at 3:00 a.m. and a peak in the midafternoon. That such a pattern had some intrinsic biologic rather than environmental (i.e., because one is awake, one is more active) basis is suggested by the fact that basal metabolic rate demonstrates a similar circadian rhythmicity, with the lowest levels occurring at 4:00 a.m. and a peak in the later afternoon and early evening.

In the report by Xiao and colleagues, as expected, average activity levels fell with increasing age at every time during the day (157). In addition, some variation in the circadian pattern of activity was noted as individuals became more elderly. In general, physical activity declined faster with age in the late afternoon and evening, and women who were older demonstrated a trend of greater activity than men in low-intensity exercise. Interestingly, the intrasubject variability in activity during the day fell as a function of age.

A great deal of attention has recently focused on the question of whether humans, like animals, can entrain circadian rhythmicity by physical activities. In modern societies, disruption of normal circadian rhythms is not uncommon, as witnessed in shift workers, travelers with jet lag, and so forth. Evidence exists that such disturbance of normal circadian rhythms may bear risks to health, since links have been documented between breaks in normal physiological periodicity and impaired glucose tolerance, alterations in leptin and ghrelin levels, obesity, and cardiovascular disease (97). Based primarily on the animal evidence, then, it has been suggested that regular physical activity in humans at risk for circadian disruption might serve salutary outcomes by readjusting deranged circadian periodicity.

Whether alterations in physical activity are sufficient to effectively alter and correct fragmented circadian rhythms for beneficial health outcomes remains to be seen. In their review of this issue, Atkinson and colleagues concluded that, based on evidence as of 2007, "in practical terms, the substantial levels of activity needed to obtain phase shifts may not be attainable by the majority of people" (6, p. 338).

OTHER VARIABILITY

Cooper and colleagues provided evidence for non-circadian rhythmicity of activity in young children (30). Using Fourier analysis on physical activity patterns in 15 children, these authors reported that high-intensity activity occurred with significant frequencies of 0.04 to 0.125 per minute. However, in a later analysis of the same data, spectral analysis of all physical activity bouts was found to be random over a number of 24-hour periods (10).

At a meeting of the Canadian Association for Health, Physical Education and Recreation in 1971, Ellis and colleagues reported periodic rhythms in children's activity as estimated by time series of telemetry heart rate measurements (48). This group of researchers subsequently studied the activity of 16 kindergarten children in a play room using the same technique (152). Spectral analysis of electrocardiogram data indicated activity biorhythms of 40-minute and 15-minute durations. These limited data indicate, then, that biorhythms may exist for spontaneous physical activities, at least for children at play.

Genetic Influences

Any biologic mechanism that regulates physical activity should, *de facto*, serve under the direction of one's genetic complement. In fact, a considerable body of research evidence substantiates such a genetic influence, thereby serving as one of the most robust lines of evidence supporting the existence of such an activity governor. Familial aggregation and twin studies have suggested an overall heritability of around 50%. Animals can be bred for levels of motor activity. Numerous gene loci associated with activity caloric expenditure have been identified in both animals and humans. This chapter summarizes this body of evidence for a genetic contribution to the control of habitual physical activity. Recent extensive reviews can be consulted for more in-depth information (79, 88, 151).

Lightfoot provided a useful schematic approach to investigations searching to identify and quantify genetic control of physical activity (figure 7.1) (88). Here one observes different levels of research methodology with increasing specificity, beginning with epidemiologic studies and progressing with greater degrees of sophistication aimed at identifying specific gene loci linked to activity energy expenditure. In fact, in each of these categories, there exists increasing evidence for a prominent genetic influence on daily energy expenditure in both animals and humans.

FAMILIAL AND TWIN STUDIES

Not surprisingly, levels of habitual physical activity tend to run in families (72). Siblings, children, and parents often resemble each other in physical lifestyles. This does not, however, prove particularly illuminating in differentiating genetic versus environmental influences on physical activity levels. Better are comparisons of activity levels between pairs of monozygotic (identical) twins and pairs of dizygotic (nonidentical, or fraternal) twins. The

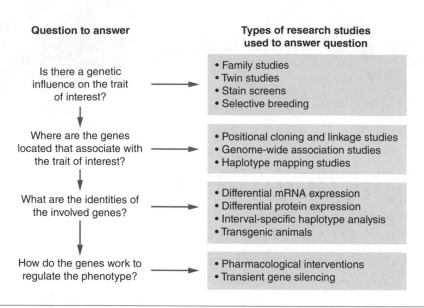

Question to answer	Types of research studies used to answer question
Is there a genetic influence on the trait of interest?	• Family studies • Twin studies • Stain screens • Selective breeding
Where are the genes located that associate with the trait of interest?	• Positional cloning and linkage studies • Genome-wide association studies • Haplotype mapping studies
What are the identities of the involved genes?	• Differential mRNA expression • Differential protein expression • Interval-specific haplotype analysis • Transgenic animals
How do the genes work to regulate the phenotype?	• Pharmacological interventions • Transient gene silencing

Figure 7.1   Suggested scheme for addressing issues surrounding the genetic basis for variables such as levels of habitual physical activity.

Reprinted, by permission, from J.T. Lightfoot, 2011, "Current understanding of the genetic basis for physical activity," *Journal of Nutrition* 141: 526-530.

former two have identical complements of genetic information, while the latter do not. A genetic influence is therefore assumed if physical activity levels are found more prominently associated between monozygotic than dizygotic twins, assuming similar environmental exposure. Based on such information, geneticists can calculate a *heritability estimate* (h^2, the extent that genetic control influences activity levels) as

$$h^2 = 2\,(r_{MZ} - r_{DZ})$$

where r is the intraclass correlation for activity for monozygotic (MZ) and dizygotic (DZ) twins. Heritability ranges from 0, meaning no genetic contribution to the variance in motor activity, to 1.0, indicating 100% genetic determination (15). As Bouchard and colleagues have emphasized,

> The environmental component shared by identical brothers and sisters may be quite different from that shared by members of DZ pairs. [Therefore] heritability estimates derived from twin data should be interpreted with caution and should be considered as upper bound estimates of the heritability of a phenotype. (14, p. 66)

A number of such twin studies have been performed relative to habitual physical activity, and they have reported a range of heritability estimates between 0.18 and 0.92. For example, a Finnish study found a heritability estimate of 0.62 for general physical activity among 1,537 monozygotic and 3,507 dizygotic adult male twins (69). Eriksson and colleagues described heritability of approximately 0.50 for total physical activity in 1,022 twin pairs, with heritabilities of 0.40 to 0.60 for specific components (occupational, leisure time, sport) (49). Among 85,000 adult twins from seven countries, Stubbe and colleagues found that 48% to 71% of the variance was accounted for by genetic factors (138). Perusse and colleagues reported a lower genetic contribution (heritability estimate 0.29) when they compared physical activity between biologically related and unrelated (adopted) individuals (112).

These studies are weakened by the inaccuracies associated with self-reports of physical activity by diaries or questionnaires and do not capture spontaneous activity or NEAT. However, two studies have used objective measures of energy expenditure in twin studies. Annemiek and colleagues examined the genetic contribution of physical activity to daily energy expenditure in 12 monozygotic and 8 dizygotic pairs of twins aged 18 to 39 years (4). Activity energy expenditure was measured by doubly labeled water over a period of 2 weeks, during which time physical activity was estimated by a triaxial accelerometer. In their daily activities, genetic factors accounted for 72% of the variance in activity energy expenditure of these subjects and 78% of their variance in physical activity.

Franks and colleagues used doubly labeled water in comparing 7-day activity energy expenditure in 38 dizygotic and 62 monozygotic twins aged 4 to 10 years (54). From total energy expenditure over a 7-day period, resting metabolic rate (RMR) (by indirect calorimetry) and thermic effect of food (considered to be 10% of TEE) were subtracted. When adjusted for age, ethnicity, season, weight, and sex, genetic factors accounted for 19% of the variance in TEE. When RMR (but not weight) was accounted for, the genetic factors explained 28% of the variance.

These numbers, which indicate a significant genetic influence on habitual physical activity, are similar to the magnitude of genetic effect estimated for other contributors to daily energy expenditure that are clearly biologically determined. Bouchard and Tremblay reported in two studies of RMR (per fat-free mass) involving twin pairs and parent–child pairs that heritability was at least 40% once age, sex, and measurement error were considered (15). These authors also found a significant genetic effect on thermic effect of a meal, with heritability coefficients in the order of 0.4 to 0.5.

This information suggests that RMR, thermic effect of meals, and physical activity energy expenditure have similar levels of genetic determinism. That is, as the major factors on the energy-out side of the energy balance equation, all would appear to be under a certain comparable level of biological control. This observation is addressed further in chapters 9 and 11 in discussions of how individual members of this triad respond when energy balance is challenged.

A number of studies have provided consistent documentation that the genetic influence on physical activity is greater in males than in females. For instance, Maia and others reported in a study of 411 Portuguese twin pairs aged 12 to 15 years that heritability of leisure-time activity (by questionnaire) was 63% and 32% in males and females, respectively (93). This information supports the contention discussed in chapter 3 that biological influences contribute to the observed sex differences in levels of habitual activity.

ANIMAL SELECTION

That rodents can be selectively bred to levels of motor activity represents a clear indication of the genetic influence on physical activity in animals. Garland and Kelly were among the first to accomplish this (56). In each successive generation of mice, those with highest wheel-running animals were mated, with progressively greater wheel-running time, peaking at a 250% increase at 6 to 8 weeks of age.

One particularly interesting observation came out of this study. The selected mice demonstrated not only increased wheel-running time but also augmented levels of motor impulsivity and overall physical behavior (45). Harkening to a discussion in chapter 4 regarding brain dopamine function and motor behavior, it has been considered that two separate systems exist— one altering general motor activity, the other reinforcing exercise behavior through a reward system. And wheel running in animals has been interpreted as a model of addictive behavior that would be generated by the latter of the dopamine systems. The findings of Garland and colleagues suggest that selective breeding increased phenotypic expression of *both* systems, implying that similar genetic influences are operant for these different types of motor activity in animals.

Such genetically hyperactive animals have served in several studies examining determinant factors associated with increased animal physical activity. For example, one can recall the studies noted in chapter 4 in which alterations in dopamine receptors in the brain have been reported in mice selectively bred for high activity levels (i.e., reference 17). As Eisenmann and Wickel pointed out, "this model may prove particularly useful for understanding the basis of physical activity since psycho-social and built environment components are all but removed as factors that influence physical activity behavior" (45, p. 263).

GENETIC MARKERS

No single physical activity gene exists. Instead, physical activity behavior is expected to be the phenotypic expression of the collective contribution of multiple genes; that is, physical activity is polygenic. Dramatic advances in molecular genetics have provided tools for uncovering these genetic factors underlying activity energy expenditure. Using innovative techniques such as genetic linkage maps, gene transfer experiments in transgenic animals, inactivation of genes (knockout mice), and identification of DNA sequence variations (SNPs, or single-nucleotide polymorphisms), researchers have provided abundant evidence that genetic loci contribute to daily energy expenditure in both animals and humans.

Several linkage studies have indicated regions of chromosomes responsible for the increased activity in selectively bred hyperactive mice (71, 89, 99). However, the effects of these quantitative trait loci on the variability of motor activity have ranged from only 7% to 17%, causing Kelly and Pomp to conclude that these low percentages indicate "the presence of a complex genetic architecture for voluntary activity likely involving many genes with relatively small effects" (72, p. 350).

As of 2014, linkage studies indicated a significant association between genetic regions and physical activity in nine studies of human beings (79). There have also been 15 candidate genes associated with daily physical activity. These include the calcium receptor gene (*CASR*), leptin receptor gene (*LEPR*), dopamine 2 receptor gene, aromatase gene, angiotensin-converting enzyme gene, and melanocortin-4 receptor gene (see ref. 40 for study citations). DeMoor and colleagues studied the association with genetic variants (SNPs) with self-reported leisure time behaviors in 1,644 Dutch and 978 American subjects (40). Thirty-seven novel SNPs were detected in the *PAPSS2* gene that were related to exercise participation. However, the associations previously reported were not confirmed.

From a meta-analysis, Viggiano identified 54 genes whose mutations produced increased motor behavior in animals but only 26 that led to hypoactivity (149). He also noted in his literature review that 12 different brain lesions have been reported to increase activity, while only 4 have diminished motor behavior. From these observations, he hypothesized that (a) a central nervous system controller may serve to continuously inhibit an intrinsically high tone of physical activity, and (b) this brain regulator of activity is sensitive to perturbations by chemical, physical, and genetic influences. Furthermore, he contended that "the hyperactivity deriving from the stimulation of dopamine, histamine, and orexin systems is in agreement with the view that these subcortical systems are 'activating' systems"

(p. 8). Such a concept of an intrinsic hyperactive state is not without precedent in human physiology. The natural intrinsic firing rate of the sinus node of the heart of a young man is approximately 35 bpm faster than the normal observed resting pulse rate due to suppression of the node by parasympathetic tone (98).

EPIGENETIC INFLUENCES

Although one's genes, the aggregate DNA complement in each cell, provide the blueprint for human life, it has become clear that epigenetic factors can control how those genes are expressed (25). Such factors may be environmentally induced, providing a mechanism by which early-life exposures can mold gene action. Moreover, it is possible for such effects of modifying factors to be transmitted from one generation to the next. A number of such biochemical influences have been identified, most common the inhibitory process of methylation of DNA strands.

Most research attention has focused on identifying epigenetic changes as a response to both acute bouts of physical activity and exercise training, offering an explanation for salutary health outcomes of regular physical activity (127). Some evidence exists as well that epigenetic factors might regulate gene influence on levels of habitual physical activity. Zhang and others examined DNA methylation related to physical activity levels measured by accelerometer in 45- to 75-year-old subjects (160). Those who engaged in physical activity 26 to 30 minutes per day had significantly higher levels of genomic methylation than those with activity less than 10 minutes per day. With multivariate adjustment, however, the significance of those group differences disappeared.

In a study comparing genetically selected high- and low-active mice, chromosome loci responsible for group differences in motor activity levels were masked by influence of grandparent genetic origin, "indicating that epigenetic interactions can play an important role in the identification of behavioral [gene loci] and must be taken into consideration when applying behavioral genetic strategies" (103, p. 176).

The understanding of the role of epigenetic factors on human behavior is very much in its infancy. Information to date, however, suggests that such extrachromosomal influences may bear significant importance. Specifically, recognizing the potential for epigenetic control of gene expression in assessing genetic–environment interactions may be critical to understanding physical activity behavior.

To underscore a point made earlier, it should be recognized that evidence for genetic control of physical activity strongly supports, but does not necessarily imply, the existence of a central nervous system controller of physical activity in human beings. Gene action plays a role in personality (energetic or laconic), psychological traits (such as level of self-image), somatotype (endomorphic or ectomorphic), and abilities in motor performance (the skilled will prefer to exercise). All of these biologically influenced factors might be expected to contribute to habits of physical activity, independent of a central control mechanism.

Physical Activity Play

D evelopmental psychologists have long struggled to find a common understanding of the nature and reason for physical activity play. Even agreeing on a definition has proven challenging. Certainly play involves acts such as running, climbing, and chasing. For sure, it is enjoyable and not serious. Play is spontaneous, free, pleasant, and voluntary. It may involve games, even with rules, and can sometimes be symbolic of more significant activities (e.g., war). In the end, one's idea of play is a subjective one. Yet, despite the lack of an official definition, every reader of these words has a clear image of the rough-and-tumble action of 4-year-olds at play.

The large volume of research on play has, nonetheless, provided some points of common ground with which experts are in accord:

• Play is uniquely a feature of the young. In what has been described as "an inverted-U developmental course," play behavior in human beings starts in infancy, peaks during childhood, and then declines in adolescence (11, p. 579). Adults do not play, at least not in the same context of kinds of behavior described here. The same pattern of play behavior with age is observed in animals as well.

• Males engage in rough-and-tumble physical play to a greater extent than females at all ages. This sex difference appears to be independent of cultural setting and is observed in animals as well. However, Panksepp and colleagues have contended that with respect to its biological explanation, "the issue of sex differences must remain an open issue. This is because the focal-observation procedure in which sex differences have been noted cannot adequately exclude the role of accruing social learning as well as other intrinsic confounds" (110, p. 470). They note, for instance, that testosterone in males triggers increases in muscle mass, which could provide a physical advantage leading to greater physical play. These authors have also made the intriguing observation that they "have occasionally observed robust sex differences in rat play experiments conducted in relatively noisy undergraduate laboratory classes, leading to the possibility that females are more readily diverted away from ludic behaviors by external stimuli" (p. 471).

• Play is an important physical drive. Children and young animals deprived of play will compensate later by increasing play activities.

• Physical play is ubiquitous in the higher members of the animal kingdom. (Indeed, entire books have been devoted to this subject [2, 50].) Bear cubs, kittens, and human children all chase each other, wrestle, and explore.

This latter observation has proven to be particularly pertinent as the basis for the expectation that physical play has a biological basis—both from the standpoints of deterministic mechanisms and evolutionary-based purpose. In this way, the nature of physical play bears striking parallels to that of the daily level of physical activity that is the focus of this book. In fact, it is not unreasonable to expect that similar determinants and rationales might be in force for both and that play contributes to the overall activity energy expenditure of physical activity. On the other hand, the temporal pattern of physical activity play, being restricted to the young, clearly distinguishes this activity from the construct of habitual physical activity. Thus, although the two forms of activity might share a biological basis, their underlying determinants and *raison d'être* are presumably distinctive.

FUNCTION OF PHYSICAL PLAY

Play has been described as purposeless, which immediately poses a problem: If play is without purpose, is one to believe that is has no biological function (111)? And why would a purposeless endeavor be observed so commonly throughout the animal kingdom? Indeed, except for the common supposition that physical play is, in some fashion, functional, little agreement has been achieved on the nature of that purpose.

This uncertainty regarding the function of physical play is reflected in the multitude of reasons that have been offered. Pellegrini and Smith have outlined the most common of these proposed explanations for the role of physical play (111):

• Since play is restricted to the young, it may provide some future benefit in adulthood. It may, for example, constitute a sort of rehearsal for activities, such as physical aggression that have a more serious meaning later in life.

• Since play is restricted to the young, it may provide some immediate benefit during childhood. Motor activity expressed in play behavior has been considered important for cognitive development of children. In animal species, temporal aspects of play have corresponded closely to certain neurophysiological events, particularly formation of synapses within the cerebellum, suggesting a more specific neurologic effect of play (22).

• Play is a form of physical training, serving to promote muscle development, coordination, and motor skills. It has been pointed out, however, that it is difficult to reconcile this concept with the age specificity of play (that is, why would it diminish during late childhood?). Moreover, the forms, intensity, and duration of activities involved in physical play do not largely mimic those recognized to cause such improvements in fitness (22).

• Physical play is meant to maintain energy and thermal balance. Specifically, such play functions to blow off surplus energy. Play behavior has been noted to decrease in animals after a period of food deprivation, and similar observations have been made in humans.

• Animals (and humans) need to maintain a certain level of stimulation within the central nervous system. Physical play acts to sustain such a state of arousal.

• Play serves as an early physical vehicle for social dominance to be expressed later in life. Taylor reported in a longitudinal study of male rats that those who demonstrated the greatest fight play as juveniles became the most aggressive adults (140).

While all these explanations might seem to bear some degree of credibility, for the most part, they are not entirely consistent with the recognized features of physical play, namely, its exclusivity in the young as well as sex-related differences. Moreover, they fail to account for the compulsive, almost addictive nature of play. In sum, then, none of these interpretations of the function of play is entirely satisfying.

NEUROLOGICAL BASIS

Although it is generally agreed that physical activity play is a fundamental neurobehavioral process, little research has been performed to delineate its neurologic basis, and information available is almost entirely in animal models. The basic drive for play behavior appears to originate in primitive parts of the brain, since play persists in animals after removal of the cerebral cortex. A number of pharmacologic agents and experimentally induced lesions have been demonstrated to either increase or diminish play activity in rodents (110). For example, diminished play behavior is observed after aspirative removal of the caudate as well as with lesions of the lateral hypothalamus. In general, play behavior is reduced by central nervous system stimulants such as catecholamines.

As Panksepp and others have cautioned, however, care needs to be taken in the interpretation of such reports:

> There is presently no compelling reason to believe that any of these studies has highlighted important attributes of play circuits in the brain [since] these effects may simply be reflections of more global behavioral changes. Behavioral specificity of changes observed must be evaluated for meaningful conclusions to be derived. (110, p. 477)

The best evidence for a true influence on a neurochemical mechanism regulating play would be expected to come from establishing the capacity of an agonist and its antagonists to alter physical play in opposing directions. Two such neurochemical systems satisfying this criterion that demonstrate robust evidence for altering play behavior in mice have been identified (110). The administration of morphine commonly augments play behavior in rodents, while opiate antagonists, such as naloxone, block this effect (figure 8.1). At certain doses, nicotine reduces play in experimental animals, while its antagonist, mecamylamine, has been observed to not only increase play but also inhibit the hypoactive effects of administered nicotine.

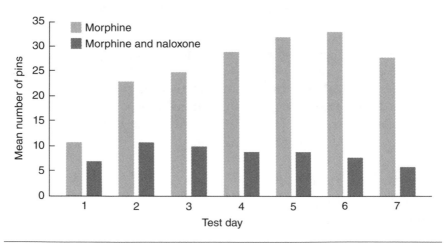

Figure 8.1   Effects of morphine and naloxone (a morphine antagonist) on pinning behavior (an expression of aggressive play activity) in rats. Increases in activity after an injection of morphine are blocked by naloxone but unaffected by a placebo saline injection.

Data from Panksepp, Siviy, and Normansell 1984.

PART II

Rationale and Mechanisms

The collective evidence provided in part I offers a compelling argument for the existence—at least in some form—of a central biologic controller of habitual physical activity in human beings. But why should such an involuntary governor exist? Part II addresses a plausible hypothesis: There is a need for central regulation of physical activity in human beings that lies in the evolutionary-based requirement for the maintenance of body energy balance. The chapters that follow examine data that are (and are not) consistent with this proposal, how temporal trends during the growing years stress the energy balance equation, and the potential mechanisms by which a biologic regulator might operate.

Activity Regulation and the Need for Energy Balance

In the realm of biology, the explanations for structural and functional phenomena are expected to be couched in terms of Darwinian natural selection. Compared to the strictly defined behavior of the macroscopic physical world (26), the predictability and precision of the physiological and functional activities of living beings are not often ensured (65). Still, in the concept of natural selection, biologists receive an over-encompassing and enduring principle by which biological phenomena can be explained.

In a schema that is at the same time both simple and elegant, Darwin wrote that within a population, variants in anatomy and function arise (now recognized as due to spontaneous gene mutations). When challenges to survival are confronted by the population, only those variants that offer advantages to survival and reproduction will persist. Biologists therefore view any particular physiologic process or anatomic structure as an *outcome*, the result of millions of years of not trial and error but rather a process of error and trial. The *errors*, the variability in biologic processes created by gene mutations, are placed on trial, and they persist if a greater opportunity for reproductive survival is achieved.

Within this Darwinian context, the proposal that an explanation for the existence of biological control of daily activity energy expenditure rests in its contribution to the regulation of energy balance and the stability of weight and composition bears credibility for several reasons:

1. Tight control of energy balance itself, the matching of energy in to energy out, represents that an important biological drive can be assumed since it *de facto* exists and, moreover, resists perturbation. Natural mechanisms, it can be assumed, do not exist for nonsensical reasons.

2. Energy expenditure through physical activity is a significant contributor in the energy balance equation.

3. The other major determinants of energy balance (i.e., caloric intake, thermic effect of eating, and basal metabolic rate) are clearly of biological origin, governed by subconscious processes.

4. When expressed relative to body size, the values of each of these variables decline during the course of a lifetime, paralleling a fall in activity energy expenditure.

Moreover, each of these contributors is observed throughout the animal kingdom, strongly suggesting that the establishment of energy balance by such variables has a primitive evolutionary origin. The next four sections examine each of these points in more detail.

By this proposed rationale, then, biologic regulation of activity as a means of establishing energy balance joins a long list of similarly controlled homeostatic processes within the central nervous system that are essential to life, such as those that maintain stability of body temperature, glucose level, blood pH, and fluid balance. That is, the concept of regulation of activity energy expenditure for the sake of establishing energy balance is congruent with the need to maintain stability of the *milieu intérieur,* the term proposed by the 19th century physiologist Claude Bernard to mean that the internal environment must be maintained within narrow physiologic limits to permit survival:

> [The human organism] must be so perfect that it can continually compensate for and counterbalance external variation. . . . Compensation [must be] established as continually and exactly as if by a very sensitive balance. . . . All the vital mechanisms, varied as they are, have only one object: that of preserving constant the conditions of life in the *milieu intérieur.* (10, foreword)

The evolutionary pressures responsible for the regulation of physical activity should not be confused with those responsible for physical fitness. Physical fitness proffered survival value to early hominids by providing a more effective means of obtaining food, escaping enemies, and avoiding environmental extremes. Regulation of physical activity is proposed to contribute to energy balance through activity energy expenditure. It is tempting to consider that physical fitness and habitual physical activity both might share the effect of a common evolutionary pressure since both involve muscular activity (63). Still, evidence indicates that physical fitness and physical activity evolved independently. This includes the observation that current literature suggests a weak or nonexistent relationship between exercise capacity among individuals and their levels of daily physical activity (63).

As has commonly been noted, it is interesting that both of these forms of motor function—performance capacity and habitual activity—have outlived their original evolutionary purpose. No longer does one need to be physically fit to obtain food and shelter, and "we may be biologically equipped for a physically active lifestyle, while cultural circumstances permit and reinforce an inactive alternative" (69, p. 375). Yet, intriguingly, in contemporary advanced societies, enhancement of both fitness and activity offer health and survival benefits, but these benefits are different from those that evolutionary pressures originally defended.

ENERGY BALANCE AS A BIOLOGICAL NEED

Objectively, energy balance is recognized to be maintained within very narrow limits (51). The outcome measure—body weight—demonstrates marked stability of day-to-day measurements, and even the observed degree of short-term variability may be attributed largely to shifts in body water content. The normal variation in an adult individual's weight is typically about 0.5% over periods of 6 to 10 weeks (54). Goodner and Ogilve reported that body weight in subjects with diabetes mellitus varied by only 3.7% to 4.6% over a period of 5 years (40).

Evolutionary selection pressure that established such a tight control over energy balance is presumably rooted in the need to prevent excesses of weight loss and gain that would occur in the absence of such control. Loss of energy substrate for locomotion and muscular wasting, on one hand, and obesity, on the other, would have been unsupportable under the living conditions of early humans.

The importance of such control over energy balance is underscored by a consideration of the outcomes if such tight control did not exist. Assuming a daily need to match 2,500 kcal food intake with a similar amount of energy expenditure, what would be the outcome if the error in doing so were ±10%? The traditional calculation goes like this: This degree of mismatch would mean a gain or deficit of 250 kcal over a 24-hour period, 1,750 kcal per week, 7,000 kcal per month, and almost 100,000 kcal per year. This equates to a yearly gain or loss of approximately 67 lb (30 kg) if the change were of the amount of body carbohydrate stores or muscle protein and 30 lb (14 kg) if by alteration in fat content.

Tam and Ravussin contended, however, based on the calculations of Alpert (2), that this type of static calculation provides fallacious results. What is ignored, they claim, is the factor of time, and the calculations should be based on a more appropriate equation:

$$\text{Rate of change of energy stores} = \\ \text{rate of energy intake} - \text{rate of energy expenditure}$$

Further, Tam and Ravussin state the following:

> This equation explains why small positive changes in energy balance cannot lead to large weight increases over a number of years. After short periods of positive energy balance, energy stores as fat mass and fat-free mass will increase and cause an increase in energy expenditure which will negate the increased energy intake. The individual will once again be in energy balance, but with a higher energy intake, higher energy expenditure, and higher energy stores. (110, p. 156)

Both of these approaches to understanding the magnitude of weight outcomes with energy imbalance are probably simplistic. Many other factors are presumed to be involved as well, such as the decrease in physical activity energy expenditure that can be expected in those who gained body fat as well as the unique balance effects of specific nutrients (110). Energy balance is a truly complex process that is poorly understood despite a great deal of research effort. It is sufficient to make the point here, though, that close regulation of body energy balance is critical, and even small errors in such control can be consequential.

ROLE OF PHYSICAL ACTIVITY IN ENERGY BALANCE

Table 9.1 outlines the contributors to both sides of the energy balance equation. Caloric intake is the sole determinant on the intake side, while multiple factors expend energy on the expenditure side of the equation. Among these factors, basal metabolic rate, spontaneous physical activity, and voluntary physical activity account for the majority of energy expenditure; the contribution of the other components is very minor. The magnitude of caloric expenditure by thermogenesis of eating is dictated by content and volume of dietary intake, and is assumed to typically account for 10% of energy out. During childhood and adolescence, caloric

Table 9.1   Contributors to Energy Balance

Energy in	Energy out
Dietary food intake	Basal metabolic rate
	Spontaneous physical activity
	Voluntary physical activity
	Thermogenic effect of food
	Growth
	Fecal fermentative gas
	Energy of urine
	Thermoregulation

needs for growth approximate 1% to 2%. The relative contributions of the major determinants of energy expenditure, basal or resting metabolic rate, spontaneous physical activity (NEAT), and voluntary physical activity demonstrate considerable interindividual variability, as illustrated by the findings in the following studies. Specifically, the relative contribution of locomotor activity to energy out is directly related to the level of physical activity.

In a seminal investigation, Ravussin and colleagues measured rates of energy expenditure in 177 adult subjects by indirect calorimetry over 24-hour periods in a respiratory chamber (88). The participants in this study, who ranged in age from 21 to 64 years, were not allowed vigorous activity but had access to television and radio, desk, chairs, and a bed. The study conditions, then, mimicked a sedentary existence without voluntary physical activity, and all physical activity might be considered to reflect NEAT. Time spent in physical activity, as estimated by a radar system and wrist motion sensor, averaged 8.7% of the 14-hour period. In this study, the total daily energy expenditure averaged $2,292 \pm 420$ kcal·d^{-1}. Average spontaneous physical activity accounted for 348 kcal·d^{-1}, or 15% of the total. Thermic effect of food, calculated as the difference between resting energy expenditure and basal metabolic rate over 15 hours, averaged 165 ± 155 kcal·d^{-1}, or 7.0% of ingested calories. Basal metabolic rate varied widely, from 1,102 to 2,935 kcal·d^{-1}, with an average of $1,813 \pm 363$ kcal·d^{-1} (79% of total energy expenditure). All these measures of energy expenditure were closely related to body weight and fat-free mass (FFM) by correlation coefficients of 0.67 to 0.71.

Schulz and others performed a study using the same methodology to determine if these variables of energy balance would be affected by high aerobic fitness in endurance-trained men (101). In this investigation, again, only spontaneous activity was permitted during the testing period in the respiratory chamber. Average measures of total daily energy expenditure (2,126 kcal), BMR (1,808 kcal), thermogenic effect of food (TEF) (25 kcal), and NEAT (289 kcal) were not significantly different from those of nonathletic control subjects. In this study, NEAT accounted for 13.6% of energy expenditure.

The same group of investigators then reported findings in a similar study involving nine elite female distance runners (average $\dot{V}O_2$max 66 ± 4 ml·kg^{-1}·min^{-1}) (100). In addition to sedentary measurements in a respiratory chamber, voluntary exercise energy expenditure involving an average of 10 mi (16 km) of running per day was assessed by the doubly labeled water method. Training energy expenditure (1,087 ± 244 kcal·d^{-1}) was calculated from the difference of free-living expenditure and that in the respiratory chamber, corrected for the thermic effect of food. In these athletes, physical activity averaged 47% of daily energy expenditure.

At the extreme end of the exercise scale, Saris and colleagues calculated daily total energy expenditure in five cyclists competing in the Tour de France (96). They calculated energy cost of cycling using a validated formula that considered factors such as cycling speed and time, change in altitude, air and rolling resistance, posture, pavement, and weight and height of the cyclist. Over 22 days of competition, the average energy expenditure was estimated to be 25.4 ± 1.4 MJ·d^{-1} (6,068 kcal), while the peak value obtained during a day of mountain climbing was 32.7 ± 1.6 MJ·d^{-1}.

Using values for basal metabolic rate and NEAT obtained in the study in endurance athletes by Schulz and others in male endurance athletes, and accounting for 10% from thermic effect of eating, the average additional daily energy expenditure from cycling the Tour de France approximated 3,800 kcal. This information indicates that daily activity energy expenditure in healthy adult men can range from about 300 kcal as NEAT in the most sedentary to 4,200 kcal (combination of voluntary and involuntary activity) in those performing "really on the edge of the human endurance capacity" (96, p. S29). In the former, activity energy expenditure accounted for 14% of total expenditure, while in the cyclists, that contribution increased to 70%. In general populations, it is usually considered that resting metabolic rate accounts for 60% to 75% of daily energy expenditure, physical activity 15% to 30%, and thermic effect of food 10% (84).

These studies show that, as would be expected, in more active contexts, the relative importance of physical activity to energy balance is greater. Still, even under very sedentary conditions, physical activity is still the second-greatest contributor to energy expenditure.

BIOLOGIC ORIGIN OF OTHER CONTRIBUTORS TO ENERGY BALANCE

While many factors contribute to the energy balance equation, only four—caloric consumption on the in side and basal metabolic rate, thermic effect of eating, and physical activity on the out—can be considered as major players. A consideration of the established biologic determinants underlying the first three of these would suggest a similar involuntary central control of the fourth.

Caloric Intake

Caloric intake through food consumption represents the sole factor on the in side of the energy balance equation. The energy provided by foodstuffs depends on its nutritional content—carbohydrate, fat, and protein provide 4, 9, and 4 kcal per gram, respectively. In addition, the actual number of calories supplied by food is affected by the degree to which it is digested and absorbed in the gastrointestinal tract. This *coefficient of digestibility* is typically high, usually over 90% for most foods, and is often ignored in calculations of caloric consumption (70).

Caloric intake is governed by appetite, or the subjective desire to consume food. Here, there are obvious parallels to the function of a proposed biologic controller of physical activity. It would seem initially obvious that people consciously control how much food they eat; that is, eating is seemingly a voluntary, purposeful activity. One plans and cooks meals, dines out at restaurants, and gorges oneself at wedding dinners, all by conscious decision making. It is equally clear, however, that appetite is a biological function, one carefully controlled by centers in the central nervous system beneath the level of conscious awareness. In fact, appetite is an outcome marker of a complex feedback mechanism by which signals of satiety, blood sugar levels, and body composition are channeled by the hypothalamus to trigger food consumption with the objective of providing adequate energy substrate and maintaining energy balance.

A quick review of what is known about the nature of such biologic control might provide insight into the workings of a biological controller of activity, which, similarly, appears to be a voluntary activity. It has a long evolutionary basis, and it serves to trigger a physical act and maintain energy homeostasis. For further details, refer to the extensive reviews of this topic (94, 127).

Biologic Control of Appetite

Control of caloric intake involves a conceptually simple, but, in fact, extraordinarily complex feedback system whereby information regarding nutrition status is fed through afferent mechanical, neurological, and biochemical signals to a central interpretative center, which controls eating behavior by efferent pathways to maintain a certain set point of desired caloric balance. The details of this system remain incompletely understood. Most information has been gained from studies in animals, and evidence indicates that factors and processes involving control of caloric intake can typically—but not always—be considered to be operant in human beings as well.

The regulatory center for caloric intake rests in the hypothalamus, an almond-sized structure located at the base of the brain, just above the brain stem. It's part of the limbic system, which includes numerous structures throughout the brain that serve, in general, to preserve the organism from threats to survival (i.e., regulation of aggressive and defensive behaviors, reproduction, feeding, and drinking). The location and Darwinian nature of these functions speaks to the structure's primitive evolutionary origin.

Besides serving as an appetite-stat, this small multitasking body acts as the primary controller setting levels of body temperature, thirst, fluid balance, and hormonal release. Control of body caloric balance occurs in several nuclei (ventromedial, paraventricular, arcuate, lateral) located in the posterior hypothalamus, with different—and sometimes opposite—effects on eating behavior. For example, experimental stimulation of the ventromedial nucleus in a rodent results in increased or diminished food intake, depending on its specific location within the nucleus (66).

The hypothalamus, then, senses nutrition status from information provided by afferent signals and then acts accordingly to adjust caloric balance by efferent triggering of eating behavior. It should be emphasized that this center works not simply as a relay center but instead serves to integrate and interpret information (66). Within a very tiny working space is a wise controller of caloric intake appropriate for maintaining the *milieu intérieur*.

The process of hypothalamic regulation of caloric intake has been divided into short-term and long-term control. The former consists of afferent signaling of satiety after an acute ingestion of food to prevent overeating. The second involves information sent to the hypothalamus regarding body energy stores with the goal of maintaining body energy balance.

Satiety information is provided to the hypothalamus by a variety of mechanical, neurological, and biochemical means. Distention of gastrointestinal structures—particularly stomach and small intestine—triggers signals to the brain regarding food volume, bringing about a reduction or cessation of eating behavior. These signals are apparently parasympathetic in nature, since bilateral section of the greater splanchnic nerve abolishes increased feeding behavior in animals after food has been removed from the stomach (98).

Afferent Information

A number of biochemical signalers have been identified that are secreted by the gastrointestinal tract in response to the entrance of food (1) (figure 9.1). These polypeptide hormones, of which at least 20 have so far been identified, are produced locally. They activate sensory receptors in the intestine wall, which in turn transmit signals via the vagus nerve to the hypothalamus, inhibiting food intake. Included on the list are duodenal peptide cholecystokinin, glucagon-like peptide-1, glicentin, glucagons, peptide tyrosine-tyrosine (PYY), and apolipoprotein A-IV. In many cases, these agents are secreted

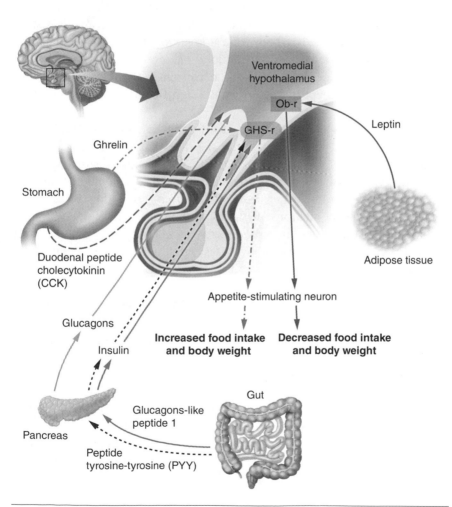

Figure 9.1 Schematic representation of factors within the gut and adipose tissue that provide afferent input to the brain regarding nutrition status in the process of appetite control.

by the gastrointestinal tract in direct relationship to the amount of calories consumed. In one study, Batterham and colleagues found that an intravenous infusion of PYY in young adults reduced food consumption by 30% when they were sent to an all-you-can eat buffet lunch (8).

Two aspects of this hormonal influence on appetite have been unexplained. First, of the large number of such agents that have been identified, all act to suppress food intake, and only one, ghrelin, is known to stimulate appetite. Second, the majority, if not all, of these agents that are secreted from the gastrointestinal tract are also produced in the brain itself.

A fall in glucose utilization by central nervous system neurons within the ventromedial nucleus may serve to augment food intake. By this mechanism, both acute threats to energy homeostasis (i.e., hypoglycemia) and those that are long term (diminished carbohydrate stores) would stimulate food intake. There is also indication that a fall in blood glucose levels causes a rise in hypothalamic norepinephrine turnover, consistent with other evidence that hypothalamic norepinephrine activity has a significant influence on control of appetite.

The lipostatic hypothesis holds that information regarding the level of fat stores in the body is transmitted to the hypothalamus by biochemical mediators that regulate appetite. Agents like leptin and insulin are both secreted continuously in direct proportion to body fat content, transmitted in the bloodstream to the brain, where they cross the blood–brain barrier and influence neurons in the hypothalamus. These agents, then, provide information regarding total energy availability in the body. Both appear to serve as lipostatic factors; that is, signaling by these agents to the hypothalamus that body fat content has increased triggers a fall in caloric intake.

The story of leptin is, quite literally, a tale of two species. Leptin is secreted by fat cells, and originally it was considered to play a key role of inhibiting food intake in response to gain in body fat. This was supported by experimental findings that animals, particularly rodents, lacking either leptin or leptin receptors exhibited voracious eating behavior. As outlined by Jéquier, in animal models, leptin participates in a three-step feedback loop: (a) leptin is produced by adipose cells as an indicator of the fat tissue mass; (b) leptin receptors in the hypothalamus receive and integrate this information; and (c) effector systems, particularly those involving the sympathetic nervous system, adjust level of dietary intake (50). This kind of information led to the hope that leptin would prove to serve as an effective pharmacologic intervention in humans with obesity. Humans, though, do not generally behave as rats, and leptin does not appear to function the same way in humans as it does in rodents. Patients with obesity, in fact, have high levels of leptin, not leptin deficiency. It has been suggested this is because leptin insensitivity in the hypothalamus occurs as a person becomes more obese (57).

Efferent Signaling and the Hypothalamus

Less information is available regarding how the hypothalamus, having analyzed the body's nutrition status, generates feelings of appetite and hunger that stimulate physical eating behavior. A number of anatomic sites have been implicated as efferent mechanisms for controlling feeding behavior, including hypothalamocortical and hypothalamolimbic projections from the hypothalamus and opioid receptor-related processes in the nucleus accumbens and ventral pallidum.

Potential mechanisms by which neurochemical mediators may bring about hypothalamic integration and command to efferent motor centers have been outlined by Lenart and Berthoud (62). These include most particularly the actions of two populations of neurons, one expressing appetite-stimulating peptides NPY and AGRP and the other producing cocaine- and amphetamine-regulated transcript. To these can be added the integrative role of melanocortin receptors, which serve to augment caloric intake. These functions are all located in the ARC of the hypothalamus and are prime candidates as primary regulators appetite behavior. From the hypothalamus, nerve connections extend to higher brain centers that can affect appetite, including dopamine centers and controllers of sympathetic nervous output.

The understanding of mechanisms underpinning the brain's regulation of appetite may be enhanced by the recent development of neuroimaging techniques. Positron emission tomography, for instance, is a method that identifies regions of increased blood flow in the brain, considered a marker of neuronal activity. Tataranni and others used this technique to assess functional areas of the brain associated with state of hunger and satiation in 11 healthy normal-weight men after (a) a 36-hour fast and (b) a liquid meal (111). Hunger was associated with increased cerebral blood flow not only in the hypothalamus but also in the insular cortex and additional areas in the paralimbic and limbic system. The state of satiation after the meal resulted in increases in the ventromedial prefrontal cortex, dorsolateral prefrontal cortex, and inferior parietal lobule.

This study also provided insights in the action of biochemical mediators. After the meal, changes in plasma insulin concentrations were negatively associated with blood flow responses in the insular and orbitofrontal cortex, while alterations in plasma free fatty acids were negatively correlated with flow in the anterior cingulate cortex and positively associated with flow in the dorsolateral prefrontal cortex.

Some have found this neurochemical feedback system to maintain a fixed-caloric zero balance to be overly simplistic. As Zhen and colleagues have commented,

> Although this circuit is assumed by many to regulate body weight and obesity within a narrow set point, much like a thermostat controls room temperature, this view has been largely abandoned in favor of a more flexible regulator that can learn from past experience and adapt to changing environmental factors (floating set point). (128, p. S9)

Among the latter, termed *non-homeostatic factors*, are "neural mechanisms of learning and memory, reward, attention, decision-making, mood, and emotionality" (128, p. S11). It does not make sense, Zhen and colleagues note, "for a hungry vole to leave the burrow if the weasel waits outside" (128, p. S10). Such observations are key to seeking insights into the etiology of human obesity, since nonhomeostatic factors controlling appetite could have a clear bearing on creating energy imbalance. As Ahima has pointed out, "Appetite is a subjective feeling of the motivation to eat. Hunger, satiety, and satiation can be overridden by desire" (1, p. 2381). Here, then, is the question, pertinent to the issue of biological control of physical activity, of the extent that conscious decision making can override a biological control mechanism. Is this, in fact, the genesis of obesity? Or, instead, do obese individuals suffer from the effects of a malfunctioning biological regulator? Or is it both? Can acute overrides of biologic control mechanisms by voluntary acts (i.e., eating that second piece of pie) cause persistent changes in these systems? Or, over time, will adaptive changes in the central regulator compensate for any such voluntary behavior? Chapter 13 revisits these issues.

In summary, control of the energy-in side of the energy balance equation—caloric intake—is governed by a feedback mechanism characterized by a multiplicity of afferent inputs that differ by nature, anatomic location, and means of conductance, providing input to a central regulator, or appetite-stat, that controls eating behavior. This appetite-stat can be, at least temporarily, overridden by voluntary, nonhomeostatic actions. Many parallels are apparent between the nature of eating behavior and habitual physical activity. This mechanism, then, might be expected to serve as a useful model for constructing a means by which a biologic controller could regulate levels of activity energy expenditure.

Basal Metabolic Rate

The *basal metabolic rate* (BMR) is defined as "the minimum level of energy required to sustain the body's vital functions in the waking state" (70, p.

105). The BMR, then, is a true baseline by which other influences on energy expenditure are added. It is determined by measurement of oxygen uptake in standardized conditions in which, immediately after awakening, subjects rest supine for 30 minutes in thermoneutral, emotionally free conditions after a 12-hour fast and no recent vigorous physical activities within 24 hours. In energy balance studies, a *resting metabolic rate* (RMR) is often used instead in energy balance studies, being more feasible because it does not require these rigid measurement guidelines to be met (usually measured in the sitting or supine position after a 15 min rest). Values of RMR are typically slightly greater than those of BMR.

BMR is influenced by several factors, including thyroid hormone, body composition, sex, temperature, and sympathoadrenergic stimulation. Most prominently among these, however, is the influence of differences in body mass, more specifically in lean body mass (as the metabolically active tissue). There exists considerable variation in BMR between individuals, and lean body mass is responsible for 50% to 70% of interindividual differences (105). Still, as Speakman and Selman have pointed out,

> Despite the large effect of lean body mass there is still a substantial residual variance in RMR. In fact, at the limits, two individuals of the same lean body mass may differ in their residual RMRs by 3 MJ/day. Since the precision of RMR measurements is about 3% (200 kJ/day) much of this residual variance is biological in nature. (106, p. 624)

In other words, considerable variation in RMR from one person to the next appears to be caused by biologic factors other than lean body mass. As noted previously, a considerable genetic effect is evident on BMR or RMR. Claude Bouchard and his colleagues estimated that 40% of individual variation in could be accounted for by genetic influences (18).

BMR and Body Mass

Changes in BMR in respect to body mass with age may prove insights into the parallel alterations in all contributors to energy balance over time, which are described later in this chapter. Indeed, temporal trends in BMR may serve as the driving factor that is matched by patterns in these other determinants. To begin, the relationship between BMR and body mass can be examined.

As expected, absolute values of BMR rise as body mass increases. The BMR in an elephant is more than a thousand times greater than that of a pigeon. But, intriguingly, BMR expressed relative to body mass (termed the *specific metabolic rate*) falls as animals—and people—get bigger. That is, the metabolic fires burn more intensely in smaller individuals. This is observed both in intra- and interspecies comparisons. As early as the year 1883, it was recognized that the relative energy expenditure of a dog that weighs 3 kg (88 kcal·kg^{-1}·d^{-1}) is more than twice that of one weighing 36 kg (36 kcal·kg^{-1}·d^{-1}) (93). The specific metabolic rate of a 30 g mouse is about 168 kcal·kg^{-1}·d^{-1}, while that of a 300 kg cow is 16.8 kcal·kg^{-1}·d^{-1}. In this case, while body size increases by a factor of 10,000, the specific metabolic rate decreases by one-tenth between the two animals (99).

When BMR in kcal over a day's time (P_{met}) is plotted against body mass in kg (M) across all animal species, the regression line descends as $P_{met} = 0.19M^{0.75}$ (figure 9.2a). When P_{met} is expressed as the specific metabolic rate (kcal·kg^{-1}·d^{-1}), the equation becomes $P_{met} = 70M^{-0.25}$ (figure 9.2b). The explanation for this inverse relationship between body mass and BMR/kg, and why the exponent 0.75 is used, has been the source of debate among biologists for many decades, with no common accord. The most intuitive explanation would hold that energy is lost from the body in the form of heat at a rate relative to body surface area. The smaller an animal (including

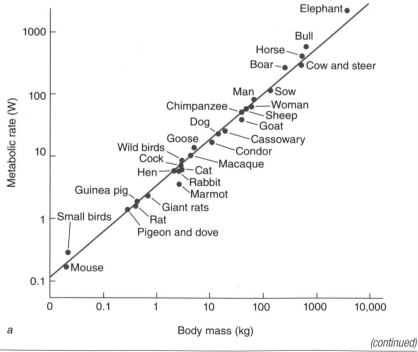

a

(continued)

Figure 9.2   *(a)* Resting metabolic rate on a log-log plot against body mass across the animal kingdom forms a straight line, with metabolic rate ~ mass$^{0.75}$.

Reprinted from Schmidt-Nielsen K, 1984, *Scaling: Why is animal size so important?* Cambridge: Cambridge University Press, 1984, pp. 56-74.

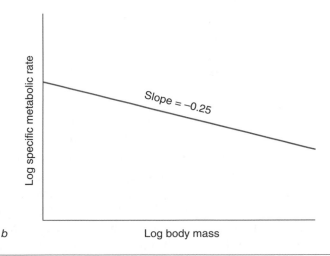

Figure 9.2 *(continued)* *(b)* Metabolic rate expressed relative to body mass (the specific metabolic rate) in the same animals is associated with body mass by the exponent −0.25.

Reprinted from Schmidt-Nielsen K, 1984, *Scaling: Why is animal size so important?* Cambridge: Cambridge University Press, 1984, pp. 56-74.

humans), the greater the ratio of its body surface area to mass (91) (figure 9.3). Thus, the mouse, as compared to an elephant, will have to utilize more energy in respect to its body mass to accommodate the relatively greater heat loss via body surface area, thereby maintaining a stable body temperature as a survival mechanism.

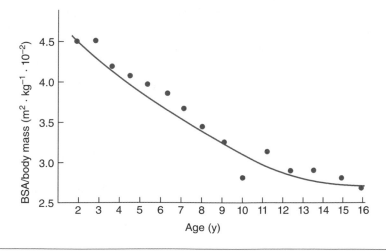

Figure 9.3   Changing ratio of body surface area to mass during childhood.

Reprinted, by permission, from T.W. Rowland, 1996, *Developmental exercise physiology* (Champaign, IL; Human Kinetics), 10.

This explanation makes sense, but if it were in fact the case, geometric considerations would dictate that BMR should relate to body mass by the exponent 0.67, not 0.75. How to reconcile this difference continues to be an unresolved issue. Many suggestions and alternative explanations have been proffered, none entirely satisfactory.

Also uncertain is whether the greater BMR/kg in the smaller animal represents a higher rate of metabolism within the individual cells of the body itself or, instead, reflects an expression of the total size of the organism. That is, either the metabolic cellular processes are more intense in smaller animals, or its metabolically active organs represent a greater proportion of body mass. The question can be considered equally unresolved.

In 1967, based on information from several studies, Holliday and others synthesized information regarding the relationship between BMR and body weight in children (48). BMR and body mass were closely linked until a mass of 10 kg was reached. Above that mass, BMR related to mass by an exponent of 0.58.

When these authors examined the decline in the combined weights of brain, liver, kidneys, heart, and lungs to total body weight as a child grows, they found similar exponents. They thus concluded that the fall in resting specific metabolic rate with age in children is a consequence of a decline in the relative combined weights of the most metabolically active organs in respect to total body weight.

In a more recent study, Butte and colleagues measured basal metabolic rate of infants and children by direct calorimetry after they woke in a metabolic room (21). BMR related to body mass by a scaling exponent of 0.40 to 0.50 in the children (ages 9 to 16 years) and 1.04 to 1.30 in the infants (ages 3 to 18 months). These findings, then, largely confirmed those reported by Holliday and others. Also, they agreed with the conclusions of the earlier study: The decline in BMR relative to weight as children grow could be explained by the slower growth of organs with higher metabolic rates (brain, liver, heart, kidneys) in respect to those with lower metabolic rates (muscle, bone, and fat). During infancy, however, growth of BMR more closely approximated that of body mass, explained by their "relative losses of extracellular fluid, increase in body cell mass . . . and compositional changes in fat free mass" (21, p. 1051S).

On the other hand, evidence exists that indicates that the greater specific metabolic rates found in smaller animals, including children, might also be explained by their higher rates of cellular metabolism. In an analysis of animals, Schmidt-Nielsen found that the mass exponents for changes in specific metabolic rate of the individual organs with increasing animal size (ranging from −0.01 for lungs to −0.30 for brain) did not (with the exception of the brain) match the 0.25 expected for the entire organism. He concluded that "we can therefore immediately see that the observed decrease in specific metabolic rate cannot be explained by the decreases in the relative sizes of the metabolically most active organs" (97, p. 91). Wang and colleagues reported similar findings, showing that the combined scaling mass exponent for metabolic rate of individual organs was 0.76, similar for earlier reports of whole-body exponents (121).

There also exists evidence in both animals and humans that the level of oxidative processes within the cell is negatively related to body mass. An inverse relationship has been found between activities of mitochondrial oxidative enzymes and body mass in mature animals. And decreases in such cellular aerobic enzyme activity have been reported with increasing age in children as well. Haralambie, for instance, described a decrease in citrate synthase activity in the vastus lateralis muscle from approximately 30 U/g at age 5 to 7 years to 20 U/g in mature subjects (42).

It is possible that both explanations are valid. In any event, the empirically derived finding is that BMR expressed relative to kg body mass or body surface area declines with age in humans, particularly in the growing years. This decline is not negligible. The specific metabolic rate of an infant is more than twice that of an adult. The fall in BMR (expressed relative to body surface area) between the ages of 6 and 18 years amounts to 19% in boys and 27% in girls (56). Although the fall in resting specific metabolic rate continues to decline (at a more gradual rate) throughout life, the most likely explanation for the rapid decrease in childhood and adolescence is the biologic principle, whatever its identity, governing the inverse relationship between specific metabolic rate and body mass.

In older individuals, in whom body size and body surface area–mass ratios at different ages are more constant, other explanations have been offered for the decline in BMR. Values of BMR remain relatively stable during the mid-adult years, but after age 50, a progressive decline has been observed (107). Fat-free mass (particularly muscle) decreases as the same time, and it has been proposed that this fall in the amount of metabolically active tissue is the major factor responsible for the decline in BMR in the older years of life. In these individuals, BMR is closely related to fat-free mass, and when Speakman and Westerterp included FFM in equations as predictors of BMR in a cross-sectional study of subjects older than 50 years, the effect of age was eliminated (107). In that study, FFM accounted for 81% of the variance in BMR.

However, Van Pelt and others reported in a cross-sectional study that RMR adjusted for FFM was significantly less in older compared to younger adults (119). This held true in both sedentary and physically active groups. In the former, subjects with average ages of 26 and 62 years demonstrated RMR/FFM values of 72.0 ± 2.0 and 64.0 ± 1.3 kcal·h^{-1}, respectively (-11.1%). In the active group, the decline was 11.4%. This information suggests that the decrease in RMR in middle and later years of life cannot be explained by loss of metabolically active tissue alone (i.e., FFM). Factors that influence cellular metabolism may also play a role in this decline.

In summary, then, during the early years of life, absolute BMR increases due to growth in metabolically active tissue, while mass-relative BMR falls because of reduction in intrinsic cellular metabolic activity and the reduction in the relative proportion of metabolically active organs to body mass. In the older years, the explanation for the witnessed progressive decrease in absolute BMR is less clear. This fall is largely the effect of decrease in lean body mass, but a decline in cellular metabolic rate may contribute as well.

This consideration of the biologic principles responsible for the effects of mass on BMR is pertinent to a discussion of function of a biologic controller of physical activity, since size-relative measures of both active energy expenditure and caloric intake progressively fall in parallel with BMR/kg. This suggests the possibility that BMR is, in fact, the driving factor in this orchestrated fall with age of the contributors of energy balance. And this would mean that, indirectly, the explanation for the decline in physical activity over the lifetime observed in both animals and humans (at least in the early years) could lie in whatever biologically accounts for the negative relationship between specific energy metabolic rate and body mass.

Use of METS for Expressing Activity Energy Expenditure

Researchers and clinicians have often used multiples of resting energy expenditure (the metabolic equivalent or MET) as an indicator of activity energy expenditure. That is, a certain light exercise might be characterized as 2.0 METS (i.e., an energy expenditure twice that of at rest), while 8.0 METS might characterize a very heavy form of exercise. Why the resting metabolic rate should be so used as a coinage of energy expenditure during physical activities is not altogether clear, since the body tissues responsible for resting and exercise metabolic rate are markedly different. Contribution by skeletal muscle, for example, is approximately 20% and 80% at rest and during vigorous exercise, respectively (70). Also, 1 MET is defined as a resting metabolic rate equivalent to an oxygen uptake of 3.5 ml·kg^{-1}·min^{-1} (equivalent to 1 kcal·kg^{-1}·h^{-1}), but it is clear that this one-size-fits-all approach is problematic. This is certainly true in children, in whom the MET concept bears little utility because of the dramatic fall in size-relative BMR with age. In adults, too, interindividual differences in resting BMR can be marked. In a review of published literature, McMurray and colleagues found that use of the standard MET definition might result in an overestimation of resting metabolic rate by approximately 10% and 15% in men and women, respectively, and by as much as 30% for some demographic groups (72).

Thermogenic Effect of Food

The thermogenic effect of food (TEF)—also termed the thermogenic effect of eating (TEE), the thermic effect of a meal, or dietary-induced thermogenesis—is defined as the rise in energy expenditure recorded after ingestion of a meal. The energy costs of food absorption, assimilation, and storage accounts for the value of TEF, which is generally considered to contribute approximately 10% to total daily energy expenditure. Individual variation in caloric expenditure by TEF is most obviously dictated by the volume and caloric content of the food consumed. The composition of the diet also alters TEE. For instance, protein triggers a rise in TEF that can be as extreme as 25% of the caloric content of the protein itself (70). As noted previously, genetic influences are also at play in establishing magnitude of TEF (18).

PARALLEL DECLINE WITH AGING

In complying with the laws of thermodynamics, energy in must equal energy out over time in order to maintain a stable energy balance. Clearly, such energy balance in the body is closely defended, since sustained errors bear potential health significance. This model of energy in and energy out has always been expressed as a static construct. It is important to recognize, as previously emphasized, that in this paradigm the element of *time* is often ignored and that energy balance needs to be considered as a dynamic process. Tam and Ravussin raised this issue in noting that the effect of changes in body composition in response to mismatches of energy balance over time might alter the magnitude of outcomes in terms of alterations in body weight (110).

The effect of time in this matching of energy intake and expenditure is also observed in another context. When expressed relative to body size, the major contributors to energy balance—caloric intake, basal metabolic rate, and physical activity—all decline with age, particularly in the growing years (92) (figure 9.4). Basal metabolic rate expressed as square meters of body surface area in males decreases from approximately 53 kcal/m^2 per hour at age 6 years to 44 kcal/m^2 per hour at age 18 (91). Concurrently, energy consumption and activity energy expenditure fall by about half (20, 52).

Here it can be appreciated that the sage controller of energy balance in the body has an additional and perhaps more challenging task. Not only must the magnitude of these factors match to create a near-zero balance, but the controller is now challenged to recognize and balance their *rate of change*.

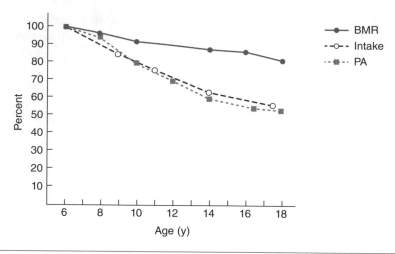

Figure 9.4   Relative decline in mass-specific basal metabolic rate (BMR), daily caloric intake (intake), and level of habitual energy expenditure by physical activity (PA) during the course of childhood.

Reprinted, by permission, from T.W. Rowland, 2004, "The childhood obesity epidemic: Putting the dynamics into thermodynamics," *Pediatric Exercise Science* 16: 87-93.

And, as in the static model, any minor error in matching the slopes of change over time of these factors will clearly result in energy imbalance. This raises critical questions: What controls the rate of decline of these determinants of energy balance? How do they talk to each other (which indeed they must)? Is one factor the primary mover and are the others reactive (it was suggested previously that perhaps BMR might a good candidate as driving factor)? Not surprisingly, the answers are yet available. Such issues are discussed later in chapters addressing potential means of biochemical communication between contributors of energy balance as they change over time as well as the implications of this dynamic model in the etiology of human obesity.

Here it is sufficient to make the point that this closely regulated pattern of decline over time in two clearly biologically regulated factors (caloric intake, BMR) is paralleled by a third (activity energy expenditure). In doing so, the tight regulation of energy balance documented as this dynamic pattern unfolds provides further evidence that this third determinant of energy balance shares biologic control with the other two.

COMPENSATORY RESPONSES IN ENERGY BALANCE

If brain centers act to modify physical behavior with the goal of maintaining energy balance, compensatory alterations in components of the energy balance equation should be expected to occur after experimental perturbation of the other determinants. That is, if caloric intake becomes excessive, levels of physical activity and basal metabolic rate should be expected to increase. If one suddenly engages in an exercise program, a rise in caloric intake would be anticipated. On careful consideration, it might be reasonably concluded that a well-functioning regulator of energy *must* work this way. If not, how can the repeated observation of a very tight control of body weight be explained?

Of course, to re-emphasize, the missing unknown element here is *time*. The central regulator may be able to accept day-to-day or even week-to-week variations in the contributors to energy balance. But eventually, over a certain period—how long is uncertain—things will even out. Compensatory changes will be made.

This is all nice armchair reasoning. Is there evidence to back it up? In fact, an enormous volume of research has focused on this issue, since it clearly has bearing on the etiology and management of obesity. Unfortunately, and perhaps surprisingly, these studies not infrequently offer conflicting results. In the end, no clear-cut patterns of such proposed and expected compensation are forthcoming. Such discrepancies have been commonly attributed to differences in study population, measurement techniques, and study design, among other difficulties in assessing the components of energy balance.

In a Consensus Statement from the American Society for Nutrition, Hall and his colleagues outlined some of these limitations that have hampered a true understanding of the dynamic nature of the many factors in the energy balance equation (41).

• The precision of measuring the individual components of the energy balance equation is low. Even the most sensitive of indicators of energy expenditure, such as doubly labeled water, has a precision of approximately 5%, which is equivalent to an error in estimating energy expenditure of more than 100 kJ per day. Whole-room calorimeters measure energy expenditure within 2%, but this is not being determined in free-living conditions. Energy expenditure estimated by self-report carries a much higher rate of error.

• Factors other than those of energy balance contribute to day-to-day fluctuations in body weight, particularly hydration status and gastrointestinal content.

• The contributors to energy balance—eating, physical activity, and basal metabolic rate—vary greatly over small periods of time. Consequently, "we are almost perpetually in energy imbalance on the time scale of hours or days . . . [and] the relative imbalance is greater over the short term than over the long term" (41 p. 991). It is therefore necessary to examine possible compensations and threats to energy imbalance over much longer periods. This is particularly a problem for balance studies performed in metabolic rooms, since humans cannot tolerate such environments for extended periods.

• Passive changes following alterations in the components of energy balance are often ignored. For example, an increase in caloric intake causing augmented body weight will automatically raise the energy cost of physical activities to move the larger body mass.

It is important to keep these issues in mind when considering the following reviews, which have surveyed published reports of compensatory changes in components of energy balance after perturbation of another contributor. Chapter 11 discusses the effect of increasing physical activity by strategic interventions on subsequent activity energy expenditure, which is most pertinent to the theme of this book. As mentioned in the preface, these findings are limited to those investigations involving nonobese individuals. A large volume of research and discussion has surrounded this issue of perturbations in energy balance, and the discussion in the remainder of this chapter, far from exhaustive, is meant to simply provide a description of trends in these findings. Additional information can be found in substantive reviews (37, 41, 46, 55).

Effect of Physical Activity on Appetite and Caloric Intake

If body energy balance is to be maintained at a near-zero target, significant increases in energy expenditure by physical activity should be expected to trigger a compensatory stimulation of appetite and food intake. This is a common assumption, one consistent with the laws of thermodynamics: If energy balance is stable, energy intake must equal energy output. It is therefore surprising that the scientific evidence, though largely weakened by inadequate study designs, has not been entirely supportive.

In 2014, Donnelly and colleagues provided an exhaustive survey of 99 published reports in the literature addressing the question of whether increases in physical activity alter daily caloric intake (32). This included cross-sectional studies of active and inactive groups, dietary intake measured <24 hours after an acute bout of exercise, and dietary changes after exercise training, both without (nonrandomized) and with a control group (randomized). Caloric intake assessment methodology varied, including food frequency questionnaires, food intake diaries, weighed and nonweighed food records, and test meals.

Among the 17 cross-sectional studies comparing physically active and sedentary subjects, 41% reported a higher caloric intake in the active than in the inactive groups. Those reports examining food intake within a day after an acute bout of exercise indicated an increase in energy intake in 23% of subjects, unchanged in 68%, and decreased in 10%. Ten studies involved an assessment of caloric intake over a time span of 2 to 14 days while subjects were involved in exercise, compared to an equal period where no exercise was performed. In these reports, half of the participants had a greater food intake in the exercise versus the nonexercise period.

Most reports have indicated that food intake in individuals is diminished shortly after an acute bout of exercise (76, 114). In a typical study, intermittent pedaling on a cycle ergometer for an hour at an intensity equivalent to 50% $\dot{V}O_2$max caused preadolescent girls to consume 700 kJ fewer calories at an *ad libitum* buffet meal immediately afterward compared to after a nonexercise session (76). The degree of decrease in caloric intake in such investigations has generally not been related to the magnitude of energy expenditure during the bout of exercise. It is likely, then, that these findings reflect a transient anorexigenic effect of acute exercise on appetite rather than a reactive adaptation to compensate for energy expenditure (15).

In a study over a more extended period, Stubbs and others measured caloric intake in six adult men who participated in no exercise, medium exercise (~1.6MJ per day), and high exercise (~3.2 MJ per day) over a period of 9 days (109). No significant effect of these exercise regimens was observed on magnitude of caloric intake.

Twelve investigations have involved an assessment of energy intake in response to a structured aerobic exercise training program (2-5 times per week), lasting on average 12 weeks (without a control group). In these reports, almost all (92%) showed no change in energy intake. In 24 similar studies involving a control group (mean duration 21 weeks), 18 (75%) failed to reveal any significant change in caloric intake, and 5 reported significant decreases in intake ranging from 200 to 500 kcal per day.

Donnelly and colleagues concluded that "overall, we found no consistent, compelling evidence that any level of increased physical activity or exercise has any impact on energy intake" (32, p. 29). A few years earlier, in 1999, Blundell and King performed a similar review of published literature regarding the influence of physical activity on food intake, with almost identical findings. They commented that "a common sense view is that exercise is futile as a form of weight control because energy deficit drives a compensatory increase in food intake. However, evidence shows that this is not generally true" (14, p. S573).

The literature regarding this issue is weakened by a number of study design limitations, most particularly inadequately powered trials of sufficient duration (32). And in terms of assessing compensatory responses for maintaining energy balance, these studies have not examined possible changes in other components of this equation that could explain failure of alterations in energy intake to match up with augmented energy expenditure by physical activity interventions. Particularly, the possibility that enhanced physical activity through training programs might initiate compensatory decreases in other forms of daily physical activity was not addressed. Investigations examining the reality of this type of adaptive change, which have revealed mixed findings, are reviewed later.

As noted previously, the time frame in which energy compensation might be affected is not clear. Certainly a short-term effect is unexpected, since Edholm and others showed that there was no clear relationship between energy intake and expenditure over several days (33). Although maintenance of energy balance is achieved over the long term, considerable fluctuations of energy in versus energy out may be tolerated over shorter durations. The studies reviewed previously may, in fact, have not examined caloric intake after physical activity interventions for a sufficient period.

Effect of Caloric Intake on Levels of Physical Activity

Less information is available regarding the effects of changing caloric intake on levels of physical activity. In animals, underfeeding increases activity. Teske and Kotz, for instance, found increases in spontaneous physical activity over both acute (24-hour) and chronic (8-week) time periods of underfeeding of genetically obesity-resistant rats (113).

Food-deprived increases in locomotor activity have been observed in rats, hamsters, gerbils, and kangaroo rats (115). Overfeeding, on the other hand, diminishes animal activity level. In one study, doubling the weight of hamsters resulted in a 50% decline in activity levels (16).

In humans, Freymond and others examined the effects of progressive overfeeding to +200% of normal caloric intake on eight 10- to 15-year-old offspring of lean parents over 3 days (36). Increases in energy expenditure, measured in a metabolic room, were small (5.9%) and appeared to be equally accounted for by changes in RMR and spontaneous activity (these differences did not reach statistical significance). Interpretation of these findings is complicated by the small number of subjects, lack of long-term follow-up with measurement of energy expenditure, and the physical activity constraints of a metabolic room. Similarly, however, Leibel and colleagues found that underfed and overfed human subjects compensated for 10% changes in body mass by altering both RMR and activity energy expenditure (61). These limited data suggest that parallel changes in physical activity with alterations in caloric intake observed in animals might also occur in humans.

Effect of Physical Activity on Basal Metabolic Rate

Basal metabolic rates measured after acute bouts of physical activity are generally elevated (75, 84, 106). This may be explained by carryover effects, such as sympathetic stimulation and hyperthermia, that are exercise induced and that persist in the recovery period. Values for BMR in those engaged in chronic exercise (i.e., sport training) would be expected to better serve as an indication of compensatory change in these two measures of caloric expenditure. Even more advantageous are studies assessing trends in BMR *during* a course of fitness training. Obviously in assessing any compensatory relations between BMR and activity, alterations in caloric expenditure need to be considered.

EPOC

It has long been recognized that an elevation of energy expenditure, measured as excess postexercise oxygen consumption (EPOC), continues to be evident after cessation of an acute bout of physical exercise. This postexercise energy expenditure has been divided into two categories based on length of duration and degree of dependence on exercise intensity or duration. Both have been regarded as explained by (a) recovery processes after exercise designed to repay energy debt (i.e., resynthesis of ATP) as well as (b) elevations in body temperature and (c) the persistence of sympathoadrenergic influences. Binzen and others reported that metabolic rate immediately after exercise was linked to blood lactate levels, suggesting the influence of anaerobic metabolism (12).

The fast component is relatively brief, lasting for not more than about 2 hours, and is independent of intensity and duration of the previous exercise. In the studies by Binzen and others (12) and Melby and colleagues (73, 74), the magnitude of excess postexercise consumption at 2 hours postexercise ranged from 7.0% to 18.6% of nonexercise control subjects.

A slow component of elevated metabolic rate after acute exercise persists from 10 to 90 minutes, and it is directly influenced by the intensity and duration of the preceding bout of exercise. Bahr and colleagues demonstrated a linear relationship between oxygen uptake at 12 hours after exercise at an intensity equivalent to 70% $\dot{V}O_2$max when exercise lasted 20, 40, and 80 minutes (4). Poehlman and others failed to observe any rise in resting metabolic rate 24 and 48 hours postexercise when the work intensity was limited to 50% of $\dot{V}O_2$max lasting for 90 minutes (85).

In some cases, even longer periods of elevated $\dot{V}O_2$ have been recorded, termed by some authors as the "ultraslow post-exercise metabolic rate" (75, p. 76). In 1935, for example, Edwards and colleagues found that football players demonstrated a 15% average increase in $\dot{V}O_2$ in the 15 hours after a game (34). More recent investigations have confirmed these longer elevations of metabolic level after bouts of acute exercise (11, 30, 31, 68). Typically, these increases are of the magnitude of 5% to 10% above control levels and are no longer evident 72 hours postexercise. In a group of 9 untrained male subjects, for example, Dolezal and colleagues reported EPOC of 24.7% above baseline values at 24 hours postexercise, 16.8% at 48 hours, and 0% at 72 hours (31).

Effect of Training

As noted before, EPOC is considered to reflect a persistence of physiologic responses to the preceding acute bout of exercise. Consequently, it would seem to have little bearing on questions of compensatory energy expenditure within the energy balance equation. More specific to this issue should be the effects of increases in physical activity, as with sport training, on resting metabolic rate, with RMR measured at a time after an acute exercise bout sufficient for avoiding contamination by the processes that dictate EPOC.

Cross-sectional studies have consistently indicated that RMR of trained athletes is significantly greater on the order of 5% to 20% when compared to that of nonathletic individuals.

Sjödin and colleagues compared values of BMR in eight highly trained cross-country skiers measured at least 39 hours after a training session with those of untrained control subjects (104). The BMR of the skiers was 13% and 16% greater than controls when related to fat-free mass and combined fat-free and fat mass, respectively. The authors proposed several possible explanations for these findings, including a prolonged persistence of acute effects from previous training bouts, a high caloric intake on days free of training mileage, or the influence of a high level of energy flux in training athletes. Particularly important among these possibilities would seem to be the first, since EPOC has been reported to persist at least 48 hours postexercise in some subjects.

Tremblay and others found that absolute values of resting metabolic rate in 30 trained men averaged 11% greater than those of sedentary individuals (117). The Y intercept of the regression equation of RMR versus FFM was higher in the trained subjects, indicating that aerobic training is associated with an elevated level of RMR per FFM. Others have reported a similar magnitude of greater RMR in trained subjects (45, 59).

On the other hand, Poehlman and colleagues could find no average differences in RMR between groups of highly trained long-distance runners who were training 100 to 160 km per week (4.1 ± 0.08 kJ·min^{-1}) and inactive individuals (4.1 ± 0.16 kJ·min^{-1}) (86). Both runners and inactive subjects had similar values when adjusted for FFM.

Could level of athletes' aerobic fitness explain these conflicting findings? Poehlman and colleagues thought so (87). They related $\dot{V}O_2$max to RMR expressed relative to lean body mass in young men with a wide range of aerobic fitness. A positive correlation between the two was significant, with a correlation coefficient of $r = 0.77$. Below a level of 55 ml·kg^{-1}·min^{-1}, no clear-cut effect of athletic training on RMR was evident. However, those with $\dot{V}O_2$max above this threshold demonstrated a 27% a greater resting metabolic rate adjusted for fat-free mass.

A single study has demonstrated that RMR falls when athletes temporarily cease training. Tremblay and others found an average 6.6% fall in RMR in eight trained individuals when RMR was determined after a 3-day interruption of training regimens (118).

Conflicting findings are also seen in studies of the influence of the training process on RMR. Speakman and Selman published a list of 11 studies that demonstrated significant increases in RMR after either aerobic training or resistance training, along with 9 studies that failed to reveal any effect of RMR with training (106) (table 9.2). None of these studies in which this information was supplied measured RMR over 48 hours following the subjects' last bout of exercise. These authors concluded that "this diversity of findings is difficult to explain" (p. 629). Perhaps the form of exercise involved as well as the intensity and duration of the training were influential. They did note that many of these reports lacked sufficient detail of study design, involved a small number of subjects, and failed to indicate when the final RMR measurement was taken in respect to previous exercise.

Three well-designed training studies are particularly instructive. Byrne and Wilmore studied RMR before and after a 9-week training program in two groups, and these results were compared with values in a nontraining control group (22). One group trained with resistance exercise, while the other engaged in a combined resistance and aerobic training (walking) regimen. To avoid the influence of EPOC, all measures of RMR were made 72 hours after the preceding bout of exercise. In the resistance training subjects, the RMR increased by 3%, but when values were expressed relative to lean body mass, no significant change was observed (−0.65%). Thus, all the rises in RMR with training could be accounted for by augmentation of mass of metabolically active tissue.

On the other hand, those in the combined resistance and aerobic training group demonstrated an average *decrease* in RMR of 3.8%. And when this was adjusted for fat-free mass, the decline was even exaggerated (−7.4%). This suggested, then, that (a) when measurement of RMR is made an appropriate interval after the last bout of exercise, the intrinsic resting cellular metabolic rate, independent of changes in volume of metabolically active

Table 9.2   Long-Term Effects of Aerobic and Resistance Training on Resting Metabolic Rate

Type of training	Reference	Time interval since last exercise (hrs) (when specified)
Studies showing a significant increase in RMR after training		
Aerobic training	Almeras et al. (1991)	
	Poehlman et al. (1990)	
	Poehlman et al. (1991)	
	Poehlman et al. (1988)	24
	Poehlman et al. (1989)	
	Poehlman & Danforth (1991)	
	Tremblay et al. (1985)	36
	Tremblay et al. (1986)	16
Resistance training	Pratley et al. (1994)	24
	Ryan et al. (1995)	
	Treuth et al. (1995)	
Studies showing no significant effect of RMR after training		
Aerobic training	Broeder et al. (1992)	48
	Davies et al. (1985)	
	Frey Hewitt et al. (1990)	
	Hill et al. (1984)	
	Poehlman et al. (1986)	
	Schulz et al. (1991)	
	Sharp et al. (1992)	36
Resistance training	Van Etten et al. (1995)	30

J.R. Speakman and C. Selman, "Physical activity and resting metabolic rate," *Proceedings of the Nutrition Society* 62: 621-634, 2003, reproduced with permission.

tissue, actually decreases and that (b) this effect may depend on the form of exercise involved in the training. In this study, RMR increased with training, as would be expected, in the resistance training group, in which responses of muscular hypertrophy are expected. This rise was entirely due to the addition of this metabolically active tissue. The fall in RMR/FFM was observed only when aerobic exercise was added.

Westerterp and colleagues examined RMR in subjects, previously not engaged in sport play, who were training to participate in a half-marathon race (124). With 44 weeks of training, total daily energy expenditure as determined by doubly labeled water rose by 30%. Over the same period,

FFM increased by 1.6 kg in men and 1.2 kg in women, but RMR (as indicated by energy expenditure during an overnight sleep in a respiratory chamber) fell in both groups. These two studies show a drop in BMR per FFM with training then suggests a compensatory response to achieve energy balance.

Interestingly, in this study, food intake (as estimated by dietary record) increased between weeks 20 and 40 in the women but actually decreased in the males. In respect to energy balance, then, the women increased calories in by food intake; on the out side of the equation, one contributor (RMR) decreased while another (activity energy expenditure) rose. In the men, both sides of the energy balance scale (caloric intake and RMR) decreased while activity caloric expenditure rose. In both groups, however, energy balance was achieved over the 6 weeks of training since, despite these changes in energy flux, little change in body mass was observed in both men and women (−1.0 kg).

Scharhag-Rosenberger and colleagues described RMR findings in 37 previously sedentary men and women aged 30 to 60 years before and after a 6-month resistance training program compared to nontraining control subjects (97). RMR was assessed by indirect calorimetry at least 24 hours after strenuous physical activity. Diet was not modified, and caloric intake was estimated before and after training. Performance on a 1RM leg press increased by about 16% with training. No significant changes were recorded in daily caloric intake. Increases were observed after training in absolute resting metabolic rate as well as RMR expressed relative to body mass (22.4 ± 3.2 to 24.9 ± 3.6 kcal·kg^{-1}) and lean body mass (29.1 ± 4.0 to 31.9 ± 4.4 kcal·kg^{-1}), but these variables were unchanged in the controls. Such differences persisted after adjustment for baseline RMR, sex, and age. The authors concluded from this information that "[although] the traditional explanation for training-induced increases in RMR is an increase in FFM . . . the present study suggests that there must be further mechanistic links between resistance training and RMR" (97, p. 1741).

Why FFM-relative RMR values should be altered with exercise training is unclear. One missing piece of information in these studies is the response of volume of caloric intake during the training period. The answer could lie in the differential responses of food intake after forms of exercise that are enjoyable and those that might be considered onerous. Speakman and Selman noted,

> This distinction does not appear to have been made previously in interpretations of the responses to exercise protocols, but it is interesting that the appetite responses of elite athletes who voluntarily engage in exercise appear to be different than those of normally sedentary

individuals recruited to participate in short-term exercise interventions. Elite athletes respond to demands by elevating intake, while volunteers in interventions respond to demands by reducing body weight and compensating other components of their energy expenditure. (106, p. 630)

The preceding studies suggest that regular physical activity might have two particular effects on RMR (106). First, with athletic training come changes in body composition, with development of a greater percentage of body mass as lean body mass, the metabolically active tissue. Second, physical activity may trigger physiologic processes that increase RMR beyond that of lean body mass, including thyroid stimulation, protein turnover, circulating leptin levels, and greater ribosomal protein content.

The potential role of the messenger agent irisin in the effect of exercise in altering RMR has drawn particular research attention. Irisin released from muscle during contractile activity may uncouple mitochondrial respiration, thereby augmenting RMR. However, this scenario of exercise → irisin release → rise in energy expenditure has been documented only in mouse models. In humans, the picture is much less clear. Studies examining the influence of exercise training on blood irisin levels and cellular actions have provided conflicting results, reporting increases, decreases, and unchanged effects, as well as considerable individual variability in irisin response (97).

Supporting an argument for an effect of regular physical activity in augmenting BMR, placing subjects on bed rest is recognized to produce a fall in BMR. A number of studies have consistently documented this effect, with reported declines in BMR ranging from 7% to 10% after 2 to 7 weeks of bed rest (13, 27, 29, 112). Whether such declines could be related to a fall in lean body mass from inactivity is not altogether clear. Molé concluded that these bed-rest findings plus the data indicating elevated BMR in training individuals "suggests that some undefined metabolic adaptation occurs with habitual physical activity" (75, p. 78). The nature of that adaptation, and any evolutionary advantage it might proffer, are currently unknown.

At present we do not know what tissues contribute to any increase in RMR produced by a single bout of endurance training or repeated bouts involved in endurance training. Further, it is not known what metabolic processes require this extra energy expenditure and what the regulating signals are. (75, p. 81)

Animal Models

Similarly in animals, investigations addressing this issue may have been confounded by different forms of exercise employed in study protocols. Most of these reports have involved forced exercise, which, as noted previously, could potentially provoke different responses than voluntary physical activities. It has been noted that RMR responses in animals participating in free-living or voluntary exercise (augmented caloric intake but no changes in BMR) are different than when the animals are forced to engage in a certain exercise protocol (RMR increases or decreases, depending on the intensity of the exercise) (106).

Still, most of the evidence supports the data in humans that regular exercise raises resting metabolic rate. In animals, Gleeson and colleagues reported that rats trained for 8 weeks by treadmill running showed a 10% increase in RMR compared to sedentary animals of the same body mass (38). A number of studies have indicated that such exercise training in animals causes an increase in resting metabolism despite losses of body mass and fat mass (5, 6, 44, 83, 126). That such adaptations reflect an increased intensity of cellular metabolic activity (rather than just augmented fat-free mass) is suggested by findings that the activity of a number of aerobic enzymes in skeletal muscle and heart are increased by such exercise training regimens (49, 77).

The ultimate expression of alterations in combined physical activity and diminished caloric intake on resting metabolism is the effect of reduction of activity and eating to zero levels that occurs with animal hibernation (108). To survive unfavorable environmental conditions, this strategy permits an energy savings of up to 88% compared to that of nonhibernating animals. In this process, normal biologic control mechanisms considered critical to body homeostasis are markedly deranged or abandoned altogether. Body temperature, for example, falls to levels a few degrees above 0 °C, and resting metabolic rate can be as little as 1% that of nonhibernating levels. Although some have suggested that the depression of RMR occurs as a direct consequence of the fall in body temperature, others have demonstrated the importance of alterations in cellular metabolism (ATP-generating systems, particularly changes in enzyme activity and function of the electron transport chain) (see ref. 108 for review).

Clearly, in hibernation there exists a shift of biologic control of energy balance to a new, extremely low steady state, one that would normally not be expected to permit survival. Presumably, this new control system is a particular sidetrack to evolutionary pressures and outcomes that allow survival in harsh environmental conditions. Such adaptations speak to the malleability of biologic controllers in adjusting to novel situations.

Effect of Caloric Intake on Basal Metabolic Rate

Following the immediate rise in metabolic rate from TEF, overfeeding experiments have consistently indicated a persistent increase in BMR or

RMR that lasts at least several days. Conversely, starvation of human beings and animals triggers a fall in BMR (78). These observations are consistent with compensatory responses for maintaining energy balance. However, it is not clear if the changes in BMR in response to under- or overfeeding reflect simply a concomitant increase or decrease in lean body mass or whether alterations in food intake can alter BMR independent of changes in body composition.

Two early investigations served as benchmark studies on the effect of caloric restriction of BMR. Both were largely motivated by a discerned need to better understand the physiologic, biochemical, and psychological effects of starvation that were commonly witnessed during the two World Wars. In the first, conducted in 1919, Benedict and others examined the effects of 120 days of a restricted daily diet of 1,500 kcal on free-living male college students at the International Young Men's Christian Association College in Springfield, Massachusetts (9). On this diet, body weight fell by 12.2%. The magnitude of concomitant reductions in BMR exceeded declines in both body mass and body surface area. Average values of daily BMR on the low-calorie intake regimen fell from 26.4 $kcal \cdot kg^{-1}$ to 21.6 $kcal \cdot kg^{-1}$ (−18.2%) and from 9.79 $kcal \cdot m^{-2}$ to 7.63 $kcal \cdot m^{-2}$ (−22.1%).

In the second study, performed near the end of World War II, Keys and colleagues recruited 36 conscientious objectors, all healthy men aged 25.5 ± 3.5 years, to undergo a 24-week program of carefully managed reduced caloric intake (53). In this investigation, termed the Minnesota Experiment, subjects consumed two meals per day composed largely of whole-wheat bread, potatoes, cereal, turnips, and cabbage. The daily caloric content was 1,570 kcal, approximately half of that consumed in a prestudy control period.

During the study, subjects were housed in a university stadium and were occupied during the day with college courses as well as with normal recreational activities. They were required to walk 22 mi (35 km) out of doors per week and spent 30 minutes daily exercising on a motor-driven treadmill. On this low-calorie physically active regimen, body weight fell in 24 weeks from an average of 69 kg to 53 kg (23.2%). Mean values of BMR declined to a level 61% of that measured in the control period. BMR expressed relative to body mass and body surface area fell to 80% and 68% of prestudy values, respectively. In respect to lean body mass, average BMR declined from 5.64 $ml \cdot min^{-1} \cdot kg^{-1}$ to 4.77 $ml \cdot min^{-1} \cdot kg^{-1}$ (a decrease of 15.5%).

These two reports, then, were consistent in respect to degree of weight loss and BMR in response to sustained significant caloric restriction. Moreover, they both indicated a reduction of BMR in excess of what could be accounted for simply by loss of metabolically active tissue (i.e., lean body mass). They supported the concept, then, that a decrease in caloric intake can bring about an intrinsic adaptation of cellular metabolic rate.

This effect of reduction of BMR after dietary restriction has been subsequently documented in a multitude of reports in both animals and humans (120). In 1995, Ballor and Poehlman performed a meta-analysis of the scientific literature to examine these results in 60 group means involving 650 subjects (6). They found that, overall, dietary restriction produced an average decrease of 12% in resting metabolic rate in these reports. When RMR change was adjusted for body weight, however, the reduction was less than 2%. These authors concluded that the reported decrease in RMR after caloric restriction could be explained simply by loss of metabolically active tissue.

On the other hand, Luke and Schoeller performed a review of studies of the relationship between fat-free mass (FFM) and BMR and the effects of this relationship with underfeeding (67). In lean adults fed a normal diet, these variables are related by the equation BMR (MJ/d) = 2.44 + 0.084 FFM. Semistarved lean individuals had BMR values less than predicted by this equation, causing the authors to conclude that the decreased caloric intake lowered BMR relative to fat-free mass.

In fact, a number of investigators have reported a decrease in BMR with underfeeding of both humans and animals that was greater than could be accounted for by changes in body weight (120). For example, using $\dot{V}O_2$ ml·min^{-1}·kg$^{0.75}$ as the indicator of metabolic rate, Ballor and others described a reduction of values from 11.17 ± 0.20 to 9.58 ± 0.23 (−10.3%) from week 2 to week 10 of moderate caloric restriction in cage-confined rats (7). With severe caloric restriction, the reduction was 19.1%. Leibel and colleagues studied the effect of underfeeding on 23 nonobese adults aged 19 to 41 years (61). With a reduction in body weight of 10% to 20%, the average fall in resting metabolic rate, estimated by oxygen uptake, was 3 to 4 kcal per kg of fat-free mass per day.

It has been suggested that such downregulation of cellular metabolism could be explained by diminution of both sympathetic nervous activity and action of thyroid hormones. Sympathetic nervous system activity is suppressed by restriction in caloric intake (58), and thyroid hormones are recognized to regulate resting metabolic rate (28). Both are recognized to be altered during studies of overfeeding and caloric restriction.

An intriguing side issue to the effects of underfeeding is the observation that prolonged caloric restriction in animals (provided with sufficient necessary nutrients) is recognized to significantly increase their life expectancy (89). This was initially observed in 1917 in rats and has subsequently been repeatedly reported in studies of a variety of animals ranging from fleas to monkeys. This effect is not minor. In a typical study, a reduction of calories by approximately 60% can be anticipated to prolong animal life span by 25% to 40%.

The etiology for this effect remains a mystery. Explanations have included the possibility that decreased caloric intake protects mitochondrial function, preserves activity of the electron transport chain, or blocks the adverse effects. It is not unreasonable to suggest that a fall in BMR in response to decreases in caloric intake might be involved, since it can be argued that specific metabolic rate (BMR per kg) is inversely related to duration of life. In mammals in captivity, life span (T_{life}) has been reported to relate to body mass (M_b) by

$$T_{life} = 11.8M_b^{0.20}$$

Previously in this chapter, it has been noted that specific metabolic rate (P^*_{met}) relates to animal mass by

$$P^*_{met} = 70M_b^{-0.25}$$

The similarity of the two mass exponents supports a conclusion, not proven, that influences of specific metabolic rate by caloric deprivation could explain extension of life span (99). That is, it is intuitive that the more intensely that metabolic fires burn, the shorter they might last.

The immediate question that arises from this discussion is whether this effect might apply to human beings (89). The question is currently unanswered, but at present it does not appear that this life-extending effect of reduction in caloric intake on animals will provide humans with hope for longer, healthier lives beyond that of preventing obesity and its complications. Nonobese humans who have restricted caloric intake for extended periods have experienced significant negative side effects (110). In the landmark studies of caloric restriction in young adult males described by Benedict and others (9) and Keys and colleagues (53), subjects experienced a variety of troublesome physical and mental disturbances, including weakness, depression, diminished libido, irritability, inability to concentrate, limitation of physical endurance, and oversensitivity to cold (they requested sweaters and stood by radiators for warmth).

Not unexpectedly, experiments in which animals and humans have been overfed demonstrate a responsive increase in basal or resting metabolic rate. Schutz and colleagues reported that carbohydrate overfeeding in humans resulted in a marked rise in energy expenditure that amounted to 33% of excess caloric intake by day 7 (102). The eight subjects of Apfelbaum and others who overate for 15 days with an isoprotein diet that included an additional 1,500 kcal per day showed an increase in energy expenditure from 12% to 29% (3). Shibita and Bukowiecki reported that rats fed an extra-sucrose diet that increased daily kJ caloric intake by 30% resulted in a rise in oxygen consumption of 11% (103).

Again, the extent that such increases reflect the addition of metabolically active tissue with overfeeding or intrinsic metabolic processes within cells (or a combination of both) is problematic. When Leibel and colleagues overfed 23 lean humans to reach a 10% weight gain, resting metabolic rate rose from $1,463 \pm 270$ to $1,610 \pm 267$ kcal·d^{-1} (+10%) (61). When expressed as kcal per kg fat-free mass, values rose from 28 ± 5 to 30 ± 5 (+7%). Neither of these changes was statistically significant, however.

The patterns of BMR or RMR with differences in feeding generally appear to indicate expected compensatory adaptations to sustain energy balance. The confounding role of parallel changes in metabolically active tissue (lean body mass) with such interventions, however, remains unclear.

Effect of Physical Activity on Thermic Effect of Eating

Since TEF reflects the energy cost of eating, the amount of caloric intake would be expected to serve as the major influence on the magnitude of this expenditure. There is evidence, as well, that physical activity may influence TEF both in animals and human beings. Two studies in rats have indicated a significant rise in TEF after extended periods of swim training (43, 47). McDonald and colleagues reported that an 8- to 10-week running training program in rats augmented TEF, but the statistical significance of the increase was eliminated when values were expressed relative to lean body mass (71).

In human studies, on the other hand, several studies have indicated that TEF is significantly lower in trained than in untrained individuals (60, 86, 116). Tremblay and colleagues measured TEF over 2 hours after feeding a 1,600 kcal meal to eight trained and eight untrained males (116). Mean value in the nonathletes was almost twice that of the trained subjects (50 kcal vs. 26 kcal). LeBlanc and others duplicated these results, finding a reduced TEF in trained men after a 755 kcal meal compared to that of nonathletes (60). In that study, postprandial plasma epinephrine levels were found to be significantly higher in the sedentary subjects but unchanged in the trained. These findings suggested that the lower TEF in the trained subjects was accounted for by their lower level of sympathetic nervous tone.

Poehlman and colleagues found that such discrepancies in TEF between trained and untrained subjects could not be explained by group differences in body composition (86). They verified lower TEF in athletes when matched with nonathletes for both adiposity and fat-free weight. The implications of inconsistent findings of TEF in response to physical activity remain unclear.

Interpreting the Evidence for Compensatory Responses

Anyone trying to draw insight from these collective data regarding adaptive compensation in the name of total-body energy balance, particularly regarding physical activity, is faced with a difficult challenge. Very few of these investigations have truly examined global energy balance, focusing instead on permutations and adaptations of individual components of the energy balance equation. In addition, frustratingly, conflicting data appear at almost every turn. As well, it must be recognized that significant confounding variables may often influence energy-adaptive studies. Before interpreting any findings in such investigations, several questions need to be asked: Was any exercise intervention voluntary or forced? Were measures of energy expenditure measured after an appropriate interval to avoid contamination by acute exercise bouts (EPOC)? Was the form of exercise aerobic, and was level of aerobic fitness of the subjects considered? Were all potential contributors to an energy balance condition included in the analysis?

An important factor often ignored in these compensatory studies is the not-inconsequential influence of interindividual variability in the magnitude and direction of such responses. The individual changes reported by King and colleagues (55) in RMR after a 3-month period of endurance exercise training in 17 adults plotted in figure 9.5 dramatically demonstrate how wide such a range can be. As discussed in chapter 12, it is just this vari-

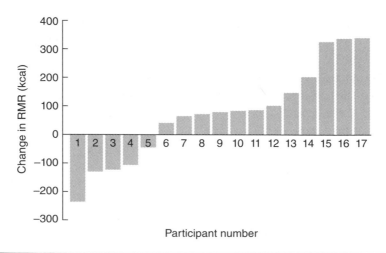

Figure 9.5 A plot of individual changes in RMR in response to 3 months of aerobic exercise training indicates wide interindividual variability in magnitude and direction.

Reprinted, by permission, from N.A. King et al., 2007, "Metabolic and behavioral compensatory responses to exercise interventions: Barriers to weight loss," *Obesity* 15: 1373-1383.

ability among individuals that may account for differences in vulnerability to obesity. As King and colleagues concluded,

> The effectiveness of exercise on weight loss is variable because individuals differ in their ability to recruit adaptive mechanisms to oppose the negative [energy balance] resulting from the imposed exercise. Therefore, compensatory responses make some individuals susceptible to weight loss through exercise and render other individuals resistant. (p. 1380)

Are there any takeaway messages? Certainly not a neat one. Westerterp made this point in an article titled "Metabolic Adaptations to Over- and Underfeeding—Still a Matter of Debate?" (123). As he commented, on one hand, "humans perfectly maintain energy balance as shown by a constant weight in adult life" (p. 443), with a remarkably narrow margin of error yearly of about 1.0 kg. This restricted variability is achieved despite (a) an enormous number of calories consumed and expended over this period (Westerterp estimated an annual energy turnover of 5,475 MJ) and (b) a considerable magnitude of day-to-day variation of the determinants of energy balance. Yet just how this stability is achieved is not at all clear from the balance data from the research literature described in the preceding discussions.

In summary, the bulk of the contemporary research literature indicates the following: No obvious effect on caloric intake is observed with physical activity interventions. At least in animals, overfeeding is observed to diminish spontaneous activity, while underfeeding stimulates locomotor behavior. Changes in caloric intake influence BMR, but whether this is simply an expression of changes in the volume of metabolically active tissue is uncertain. Studies investigating the influence of physical activity on BMR and TEF have provided conflicting results.

Because the research data do not clearly indicate a compensatory interplay between the major weights on the energy balance scale (caloric intake, RMR, physical activity), some have suggested that other more obscure, subtle effects could be at play. These would include factors such as alterations in digestion efficiency of food, muscle energy efficiency, or contributions of energy out that are missed by measurement techniques (such as NEAT). Others would point out, too, that the influence on time required for achievement of energy balance in studies of interventional effects has often been inadequately appreciated.

Mechanisms for Biologic Control

T he quest for understanding how things work has a noble history. As Carl Craver and Lindley Darden have emphasized in their introduction to *In Search of Mechanisms,*

> The search for mechanisms is one of the grand achievements in the history of science. The achievement is first and foremost conceptual: it is the very idea that scientific activity should be organized to advance the discovery of mechanisms that produce, underlie, or maintain the diverse manifest phenomena of our world. . . . The crowning aim of science is to open the black box of nature and show how it works. (25, p. 2)

Understanding mechanisms permits the ability to predict, control, and manipulate any particular process to profitable ends. Through knowledge of the operation of an automobile engine, the mechanic can identify and repair its malfunction. In recognizing why certain groups in the population are adverse to his policies, the politician can strategize to gain votes. In the present case, insight into the workings of a biological regulator of physical activity obviously offers the potential to alter any such controller to improve levels of physical activity for salutary outcomes.

The operant features of such a central governor of activity energy expenditure are currently unknown. Still, a feasible feedback mechanism is proposed in this chapter, which is based on recognized structures and functions involved in similar homeostatic control centers in the central nervous system. This includes a consideration of afferent and efferent signaling systems, a central regulatory center in the hypothalamus, and candidate biochemical agents to permit activity energy expenditure to communicate with control systems of other components of energy balance.

This chapter addresses the concepts of a proposed *activity-stat,* which would serve to regulate physical activity to a certain set point, and an *energy-stat,* an overriding control center responsible for total-body energy balance. This discussion also compares two proposed types of regulatory centers in the brain, one with a fixed activity set point and the other with a changeable set point.

FEEDBACK SYSTEMS

The mechanism behind a biological controller of physical activity, as well as of the other components of the energy balance equation, is one that serves to *maintain a state of equilibrium.* Indeed, as discussed previously, the *milieu intérieur* is preserved by means of a multitude of controlling centers functioning as part of feedback loops—incoming signals providing information regarding the status quo (a center that possesses knowledge of the proper set point for physiologic function) and efferent signals to adjust the effectors of the variable to that optimal level.

American physiologist Walter Cannon reinforced this concept in 1932 when he proposed the term *homeostasis* to describe the requirements— indeed, the necessity—of steady-state conditions in living beings (23):

> Homeostasis is the strategy, the culmination of countless years of evolution, by which the body reacts to every change in the environment with an equilibrating response. The goal of each response is to maintain an internal balance, which evolution has decided is a good thing for animals. (122, p. 38)

And so the human physiology is replete with a myriad of such controlling mechanisms for maintaining physiologic stability in the requirement for body homeostasis. Despite challenges from wide swings in environmental heat and cold, body temperature is regulated very little beyond a degree or two. Departures from such narrow control limits create risk of illness and even death. Blood oxygen content, cell pH, body water content, solute concentrations in plasma, caloric intake, blood pressure—their remarkable stability over time is maintained for the needs of physiological constancy. And all have been developed over millions of years in accord with the essential Darwinian strategy—they ensure survival.

Complex but highly effective feedback systems for such critical controls are the mechanisms that have been selected by nature in this evolutionary process. Their concept is simple. Detectors in the body sense the status of a variable (temperature, blood sodium concentration) and send this information by afferent nerve transmission to a central controlling body in the brain. This center recognizes the level of perturbation of the variable from a desired *set point* (e.g., how far is the oxygen content of the blood drifting from the required level?). To adjust the variable back to its required level, this controlling center signals, through efferent nervous tracts, the means of adjusting the variable back to the set point (e.g., appetite is stimulated to increase caloric intake if blood sugar drops to inappropriate levels).

Within this simple, straightforward schema lies hidden an extraordinary complexity of redundancy (backup mechanisms), multilevel function (anatomical, physiological, biochemical, psychological), temporal shifts, and the adverse influences of disease processes. Consequently, the details of the workings of such feedback mechanisms remain largely obscure. They work with amazing precision, but just how is uncertain.

Humans have adopted such feedback systems in building their own machines as well, like the thermostat that controls temperature in the home to a comfortable level or the cruise control in an automobile that automatically maintains a constant speed. They all mimic the wisdom of nature: information from peripheral sensors in to an erudite analyzer that sends signals out to an effecter that adjusts an outcome to a desired constant level.

One of the features of biological feedback mechanisms is that they are *deterministic*—they're hardwired into one's genetic endowment, working below the level of consciousness, and are not vulnerable to human behavior or cognitive decision making. This is not to imply, however, that the set point of such a controller is not subject to alteration by extrinsic influences and free of vulnerability to error. These aspects of the plasticity of biologic control systems are addressed in chapter 13.

These physiologic feedback systems and their set points function well beneath the level of human consciousness. One does not recognize that kidney retention of water by antidiuretic hormone is occurring when becoming dehydrated during a tennis match. Or that one needs to step up sweating rate for cooling during a 10K road race in the heat of July. But, intriguingly, certain deterministic mechanisms—which must closely regulate variables to permit homeostasis—are temporarily alterable by cognitive will. That is, their control to a set point is obligatory, yet they can, at least for a short time, be affected by one's decision making. Respirations and caloric intake are obvious examples. One can take a few deep breaths before going on stage to deliver a speech or hold one's breath during the scary part of a movie. One can decide to head out for a big meal at a restaurant with friends or indulge oneself at the never-ending buffet on a Caribbean cruise. But these apparent acts of free will on breathing and eating behavior are deceiving. They're only temporary, and a biologic controller will eventually compensate for such indiscretions, restoring a physiologic steady-state balance over time to a particular involuntary set point.

A proposed biological control of energy expenditure by physical activity fits nicely into this kind of voluntary–involuntary behavior model. Although it would appear that one elects to engage in certain physical activities over the course of a day, an involuntary governor might serve to contribute to the regulation of such activity energy expenditure over time to a particular level in the name of total-body energy balance.

Some have contended that a view of a biologic controller as rigidly defending a particular physiologic set point is overly simple. As West has noted, when one actually measures them, these outcome variables of homeostatic feedback mechanisms, in fact, do vary over time (122). The most obvious are circadian rhythms, the ubiquitous 24-hour period swing in homeostatically controlled physiologic values. One's body temperature is warmest around 6:00 p.m. with a temperature of approximately 37.2 °C. Levels then fall to a nadir of around 36.3 °C at 4:00 in the morning. Blood pressure levels are highest early in the morning on awakening. Blood glucose levels normally peak at 4:00 a.m. These regular diurnal rhythms have been observed in the functions of virtually every living being in which they have been investigated, including single-cell organisms.

Such variations are also evident over short time observations. If one records and plots a graph of the frequency of breaths, or the interval between heartbeats, over a period of 10 to 15 minutes, one observes not steady values but instead what looks like random variation. But sophisticated statistical analyses indicate that such fluctuations have a certain pattern of hidden regularity as well.

Why should such systematic variability occur? What would be its biological function? Evidence for an answer comes, perhaps, from observing the constant shift in body position of the tightrope walker. Or the variations in the motions of the magician who is balancing a spinning plate on a stick. And the minor repetitive corrective alterations of movements of one's hands on the steering wheel to keep an automobile headed straight in the lane. Quite paradoxically, it would seem, stability requires variability.

Organized variability is evidence of the presence—overt or not—of biologic control. As described in chapter 6, such rhythmic variability is evident in the extent of daily activity energy expenditure, although currently this avenue of research has been limited.

PROPOSED BIOLOGIC CONTROL SYSTEM FOR HABITUAL PHYSICAL ACTIVITY

No one has insight into the particulars of the operation of a biologic regulator of activity energy expenditure. Such a system is often highly complex and not easily decipherable. Garland and colleagues summarized this well:

> Very little is known about the neurobiology of voluntary exercise, spontaneous physical activity or sedentary behaviors in healthy animals. Various neural correlates of generalized locomotor activity have long been the subject of considerable research, but central themes are difficult to extract. In general, locomotor activity in both humans and rodents is controlled by a complex cascade of neurochemical interactions that coordinate central neural inputs with motor outputs. . . . [In addition] a litany of other neural systems beyond those required for basic motor control become relevant, including those involved in aversion, conditioning, learning and the desire for and perception of both exogenous and endogenous rewards. (37 pp. 213-214)

At the same time, it should be possible to take established elements regarding motor behavior reviewed in this book and create a simplistic but still intellectually satisfying framework by which a feedback system controlling habitual motor activity might operate. What follows, then, is this author's proposed schema—a theoretical blueprint—of the components of a feedback system by which levels of habitual physical activity might be regulated (figure 10.1).

In examining and judging this hypothetical construct, it is useful to consider what Craver and Darden outlined as the necessary "virtues of good mechanism theories" (25, p. 83):

- The theory should be able to be tested by considerations of empirically based evidence.
- The theory should be coherent and free of contradictions.
- The theory should stimulate new ideas by generating more questions than proposed answers.
- The theory should be consistent with previously recognized phenomena and their accepted cause-and-effect relations.
- The theory should be simple yet elegant.

The proposed feedback system by which activity energy expenditure might be regulated begins with afferent input to a central regulator provided

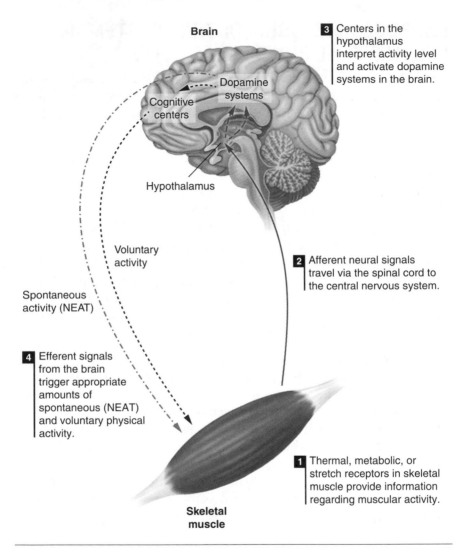

Figure 10.1   A hypothetical schema by which a central regulator of activity energy expenditure might operate.

by several peripheral sources, including metabolic, pressure, and thermal receptors within muscle tissue. Consistent with its recognized function as a feedback controller for many of the body's feedback regulatory systems, the hypothalamus serves as the central controller of habitual motor activity in this schema. Efferent output to stimulate physical behavior in response to signals from the hypothalamus occurs in dopaminergic neurons within two centers in the brain—one serving to regulate spontaneous muscular activity (NEAT), the other triggering activity by willful intentions.

Afferent Signalers

Consistent with the multitude of documented mechanisms by which caloric status is monitored in control of appetite, a number of peripheral receptors in muscle tissue could serve to assess motor activity. By ascending nerve pathways, these would provide a picture of the status of muscular energy expenditure to the hypothalamus in the brain.

Pressure and Stretch Sensors

Thinly myelinated sensory fibers (group III) innervate skeletal muscle. These are triggered by stretch and distortion of muscle during locomotion, and they provide afferent information regarding muscular activity by means of ascending spinal cord pathways to control centers in the brain (80). There this information is used to provide autonomic control of the heart during exercise, particularly in inhibiting parasympathetic activity. Most information regarding the action of these mechanoreceptors has been gained from research in animals, since deciphering their function in humans is confounded by concomitant inputs from other reflexive circuits involving both the baroreflex and central command.

Metaboreflex

Group IV unmyelinated sensory fibers in skeletal muscle are stimulated by chemical stimuli, specifically the metabolic by-products created locally during muscular contraction. The particular metabolites responsible for this neural response are unclear; candidates include potassium, lactic acid, bradykinin, and phosphates. Afferent data regarding muscular activity are relayed to the brain where an efferent response augments sympathetic activity and controls blood flow. In animals, this metaboreflex may trigger blood flow alterations in response to mismatches between oxygen supply and demand. Whether this function occurs in humans is unclear (19). Evidence does exist in humans that the metaboreflex increases systemic vascular resistance and thereby acts to control volume of regional blood flow.

Thermal Receptors

The muscular contractile apparatus functions at a low level of energy efficiency. With contraction of skeletal muscle, approximately 25% of chemical energy is converted into external work (i.e., moving a limb), while the rest is released as heat. Even at very low levels of exercise (26% $\dot{V}O_2$max), temperature in the quadriceps femoris muscle has been reported to rise 1.7 °C (95). This rise in temperature is sensed by specialized receptors to heat located not only in muscle but also in skin, subcutaneous tissue, and deep organs, as well as in the brain itself. Increasing nerve traffic from these nerve endings provides afferent information to the hypothalamus to initiate compensatory thermoregulatory mechanisms for maintaining a constant body temperature (81). Similarly, such thermosensitive receptors could provide input about the level of habitual motor activity as manifest by elevations in temperature of exercising skeletal muscle.

Central Controller: The Hypothalamus

The top candidate for the role of the central controller in the regulation of physical activity in this feedback loop by a wide margin is the hypothalamus at the base of the brain. As reviewed previously, this small structure, not much more than a centimeter in length, serves as the hub for maintaining afferent–efferent balance in a variety of the body's homeostatic mechanisms, including fluid balance, temperature, and caloric intake. Lesions of the ventromedial hypothalamus reduce motor activity in rats (115). The same effect is observed when this region is poisoned by chemical agents.

The inner workings of such a center are unknown, but it is not unlikely, as indicated by animal studies, that certain biochemical mediators, namely propiomelanocortin (POMC), which acts on melanocortin receptors, and a number of other strange-sounding chemical bedfellows (cocaine- and amphetamine-regulated transcript [CART], peptide Y, adenosine monophosphate–activated protein kinase [AMPK], and mammalian target of rapamycin [mTOR]) play a role (62).

Efferent Signalers

A biologic regulator of physical activity in humans could operate by controlling the level of spontaneous, mainly involuntary physical activity (NEAT) or by increasing motivation to participate in planned voluntary activities. Chapter 4 highlights animal studies with evidence that, in fact, separate dopaminergic domains exist in the brain for both of these types of activity energy expenditure. In rodent models, these two centers regulate volume of spontaneous activity and wheel-running activity, respectively. It has been suggested that the latter is analogous to reward-motivated behavior in humans. The critical role of dopamine and dopamine receptors in these functions is indicated by the reduction in exploratory and spontaneous activity observed after administration of dopamine antagonists in rats (37). It is reasonable to propose, then, that the efferent limb of the feedback loop of a biologic controller of activity would involve the actions of these foci of dopaminergic neurons.

Biochemical Communicators

Besides communication within the feedback system, a valid schema for biologic control must include a means by which activity energy expenditure can correspond with other determinants of the energy balance equation (particularly caloric intake and basal metabolic rate). Such communication could occur by neurologic cross-talk among the various elements of the feedback system, particularly at the level of the hypothalamus. The concept of a master energy-stat that would oversee energy balance after considering information from the components of energy balance is addressed in the next section.

It is possible, too, that extra-system exchange of information could be affected by biochemical mediators already addressed in this book, such as leptin, insulin, and ghrelin (79). Ceccarini and others proposed that animal studies supported a leptin-melanocortin pathway as the pivotal player in body weight regulation and locomotor behaviors (24).

Recent information suggests that skeletal muscle can act as an endocrine organ. That is, like the thyroid gland or the adrenal gland, it secretes circulating chemical agents (hormones) that travel in the bloodstream and affect tissue functions far removed from the site of origin. During contractions, skeletal muscle secretes myokines, and at least one of these, irisin, can influence energy homeostasis by its actions on fat cells (82). Exercise stimulates irisin release from muscle through a genetic transcriptional coactivator (an agent that acts to control gene expression) termed peroxisome proliferator-activated receptor γ coactivator 1α (PGC-1α) (64). Boström and colleagues showed that exercise stimulates the actions of PGC-1α, which triggers release of irisin from skeletal muscle, causing reduced body weight and improved metabolic homeostasis in obese mice (17). Such circulating hormonal mediators released by muscle could serve as indicators of activity energy expenditure, both within the proposed feedback schema (i.e., as providers of afferent information) and as communicators with other feedback mechanisms (appetite, BMR) within the broad construct of maintenance of energy balance.

How is this proposed feedback schema to be judged? Craver and Darden categorized hypothetical mechanisms, in descending order of credibility, as (a) *how-actually*, those that "satisfy known constraints on component, activities, and their organization with one another, and [one which] coheres with other well-supported, non-rival theories," (b) *how-plausible,* "schemas that are more less consistent with more or fewer known constraints on the components of the mechanism," and (c) *how-possibly,* which describes "how a set of parts and activities might be organized, [although] it may be unknown whether the conjectured parts exist and, if they do, whether they can engage in the activities attributed to them by the schema" (25, p. 34-35).

On this scale, this author self-grades the hypothetical construct as (b) *how-plausible*. The basic feedback mechanism is a traditional one, mimicked by a good number of other biologic control mechanisms, most notably hypothalamic control of appetite and caloric intake. The afferent and efferent components are all recognized processes; the hypothalamus as integrator of activity energy expenditure is highly consistent with its function as controller of other physiologic functions. Overall, it can be reasonably argued that the schema bears considerable credibility.

ACTIVITY-STAT VERSUS ENERGY-STAT

Up to this point, a compelling body of evidence has been set forth that a biological regulator of habitual physical activity exists in both humans and animals. A reasonable argument for an evolutionary role for such a central controller in maintaining energy has been presented, and an unproven but plausible mechanistic construct has been hypothesized. In this schema, a biologic center in the brain that governs activity energy expenditure gathers afferent information regarding level of motor activity, analyzes this in respect to a desired level of physical activity, and triggers motor activity to match this set point.

In effect, then, the biologic controller of activity premise supposes an activity-stat. Excessive physical activity would be compensated for by a downregulation of subsequent activity energy expenditure to maintain the set point, the basic construct of traditional biological negative feedback systems. The existence of an activity-stat, and of the biologic control of activity itself, would be supported if such compensatory changes were observed with exercise interventions. Consider a group of young men who are placed in a 10-week program of exercise intervention involving an hour of daily walking. One might calculate that this would increase weekly energy expenditure by about 800 kcal. But, according to the concept of a tight control of an activity-stat, this rise would be met by a compensatory decline in physical activity outside of the program, such that the actual added energy expenditure by the walking program would be minimized or even eliminated.

A good deal of research has addressed the existence and implications of a proposed activity-stat and whether such physical activity compensation actually occurs (35, 37, 39, 90, 125). Chapter 11 provides a full consideration of the research examining this question. But, in summary, these data are conflicting and are not consistently forthcoming on whether such compensation actually occurs.

Although the concept of activity-stat bears credibility, one is left with some unresolved issues. Most particularly, how does such a tight control system, limited to activity energy expenditure, work in concert with similar feedback systems within the energy balance equation to establish overall maintenance of energy balance? How could such a system of control contributing to a stable energy-out side of the equation *in isolation* work toward overall balance with other contributors that similarly appear to equally work restricted to their own physiologic domain? Caloric intake, for example, the only contributor to energy in, is closely regulated by a complex feedback system that maintains a constancy of body weight and compensation. The role of feedback loops in controlling basal metabolic rate is more obscure, but if BMR is influenced by factors other than mass of lean body tissue, this should be expected to occur. The question is this: How is cross-domain energy balance achieved?

One possible answer is the existence of a central energy-stat, operating at a higher executive level than the activity-stat and appetite-stat, which serve to control individual elements of the energy balance equation. This overseeing controller could actually exist not as a particular anatomic regulator but rather as a system of interlocking controllers that allows communication between the components of energy balance—yet still one that acts to establish energy balance to a certain fixed set point. That such a master governor exists, and that its set point is fixed, are evidenced by the observation that (a) body weight and composition normally remain remarkably stable over the long term and (b) both are stubbornly resistant to the perturbations of daily variability in energy intake and expenditure.

In this concept, the role of the energy-stat would be to regulate the set points for the activity and the appetite-stats. In other words, these latter controlling mechanisms work within their separate domains to achieve balance toward a set point, but this point is variable and dictated by the master energy-stat acting in accordance with the need to establish total-body energy balance stability. This idea of changeable or settling rather than set points is, in fact, consistent with the means by which many have considered that energy control operates (39, 41, 51).

In an ideal world, this construct would be readily tested experimentally. By altering activity or food intake and measuring reciprocal outcomes, the validity—or not—of a compensation between self-controlled domains should be evident. As the research data reviewed earlier in this chapter demonstrate, however, all is not that clear. In general, the findings are supportive of this kind of reciprocal change in determinants toward a balanced outcome. But many investigations report incomplete compensations, while others reveal findings even contradictory to expectations. It might be concluded from these observations that the construct proposed previously lacks authenticity. On the other hand, it can reasonably be argued that factors of weak research design, inadequate accuracy of measurement tools, and a failure to consider the time frame of long-term compensations might explain outcomes inconsistent with the model.

In this construct, the compensation for physical activity interventions by reduction in extra-program activity levels takes on a different meaning beyond that of testing the validity of the activity-stat concept. In this more global view of body energy balance control, any given exercise intervention could be met with a compensatory increase in appetite, decreases in BMR, or a reduction in extra-program activity energy expenditure. The absence of compensatory changes in activity itself, then, would not necessarily weaken the validity of the construct of an activity-stat working as subservient to a more globally conscious energy-stat. Studies of compensation of physical activity changes after an exercise intervention, then, would be expected to provide information not about whether an activity-stat exists but rather about the context in which it operates.

The mystery of just how stable body energy balance is established through coordinating the influences of the various members of the energy balance equation is not likely to quickly unravel. Still, it is obvious that such insights will be critical for understanding the basic mechanisms that underlie perturbations of this machinery, particularly human obesity.

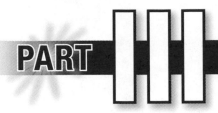

PART III

Implications of Biologic Regulation of Activity

To this point, a compelling body of evidence for the existence of biologic control of physical activity has been introduced and a reasonable rationale offered for its evolutionary-based *raison d'être*. A hypothetical mechanism for its function was then constructed based on well-established principles of homeostatic feedback systems witnessed in a myriad of other biologic controllers. The discussion in this section now turns to the issues of "so what?" Is this a fixed, immutable activity governor—like biofeedback controllers of body temperature and acid–base balance and fluid content—that operates largely at the exclusion of extrinsic environmental interventions? Or, as seems evident from our daily experiences, do the cognitive decision-making capabilities that separate human from other members of the animal kingdom provide free will—apart from any such biologic regulation—to decide how much to exercise?

Where and how does obesity—ostensibly an error in the maintenance of energy balance—fit into this discussion of biologic control of activity? Can the set point of a proposed biologic controller of activity, or that of an even more superior energy-stat, be altered? If so, is there an opportunity here for pharmacologic treatment of obesity based on a physiological rather than a behavioral perspective? All these issues are largely uncharted territory. From here on out, the scientific footing becomes increasingly treacherous, and firm conclusions are elusive. Here one enters, it might be termed, the realm of reasoned speculation.

Responses to Activity Interventions

During a routine office visit, a physician notes that his patient has jumped from the 20th to the 60th percentile for body mass index (BMI), a marker of body fat, and that he is engaging in virtually no regular physical activity. The doctor prescribes a program of regular walking, starting at 0.25 mi (0.4 km) every other day and then progressing over 2 months to 2 mi (3 km) four times weekly. By this time, he calculates that his patient will be expending about 4,000 calories each month.

What will his patient's response to such a program be? Assuming his compliance, several possibilities exist. First, the extra calories expended during the prescribed walking could be compensated for by a similar magnitude of decreases in out-of-program activity energy expenditure, resulting in no overall change in energy out, overall energy balance, or weight change. Second, adaptations might occur in other members of the energy balance equation, either fully or partially. For instance, with a fully compensatory dietary increase of 125 calories per day, energy balance would also be unchanged, with no loss of weight. However, a reduction in weight would occur if such compensatory changes in caloric intake were incomplete in matching the augmented energy expenditure in the walking program. Third, the mismatch in energy balance caused by the increased caloric expenditure of the walking program could cause a resetting, or modulation, of the mechanism-controlling energy balance, resulting in a decrease in the patient's body fat content. Finally, the exercise prescription might also trigger a long-term improvement of the patient's physical activity habits, with extended health benefits. This chapter examines each of these possible outcomes.

COMPENSATORY CHANGES IN PHYSICAL ACTIVITY

This is the originally proposed activity-stat concept: A set point for activity energy expenditure exists, such that any exercise intervention program would be met, or compensated for, by an equivalent amount of reduction of out-of-program activity and that the net change in activity energy expenditure would be zero. That is, in this response, a physical activity intervention serves to *perturb* the activity energy expenditure homeostatic system, but only temporarily, and such interventions do not act to *modulate* (change) activity behavior over the long term. Recording of a compensatory decline in physical activity after an exercise intervention would serve to support this concept. Studies addressing this idea have often focused on the pediatric age group.

In 2011, T.J. Wilkin and J.J. Reilly participated in a literary debate in the *International Journal of Obesity* regarding this question: Can we modulate physical activity in children? In the pages of this argument, they took a stand—Wilkin for the yea and Reilly for the nay—about whether activity compensation offsetting physical activity interventions was likely. Wilkin based his argument against a lasting effect of activity intervention on sustained activity habits (in youth) and in support of the activity-stat hypothesis on the grounds that (a) the research literature indicates that variations in environmental influences on young children (school physical education, geographical location) have little effect on levels of habitual activity and (b) studies indicate that compensatory declines in activity occur after exercise interventions (77). Moreover, although (c) some studies indicate increases in total physical activity after exercise interventions, there is a clear inverse relationship between such an effect of the intervention and the duration that the outcome was measured. That is, a compensatory decline in out-of-program activity occurs that acts to neutralize the effect of an activity intervention, but this may take time.

In conclusion, Wilkin contended,

> There is no evidence that we can modulate the physical activity of children, although it can clearly be perturbed. There is a danger that the success of some short term studies in raising physical activity is being misinterpreted as modulation when it is really perturbation which will last only for as long as the environmental disturbance that caused it. (77, p.1275)

Reilly countered that "the body of evidence is inconsistent with the activity-stat hypothesis in its current form and suggests that the emphasis on physical activity in obesity prevention interventions in children should be increased, not reduced" (55, p. 1266). In his rebuttal, he cited systematic reviews that indicate favorable effects of physical activity interventions and the potential for environmental manipulations to promote physical activity. The data concerning heritability he considered to demonstrate only a weak effect. Instead, he supported the role of environmental factors as dominant in influencing habitual physical activity. Reilly thought that the current research literature failed to indicate compensatory decrease in habitual activity with exercise interventions, although he acknowledged that these reports generally measured such responses in terms of days and that "compensation may occur over longer periods" (p. 1267).

It is evident, then, this controversy can be viewed from various vantage points, interpreting the same set of experience in the research literature as supportive to divergent arguments. It is worthwhile to examine some of these points of discussion in more detail.

Wilkin and colleagues presented their arguments (outlined previously) in support of the activity-stat concept, which "would comprise a neuro-humoral feedback loop, with a set-point possibly located in the hypothalamus, able to integrate activity carried out by as yet unknown means, and to control further activity accordingly. If centrally controlled in this way," they reasoned, "we would expect overall physical activity to be independent of environmental opportunity or (within limits) of environmental intervention" (78, p. 1050).

To examine this hypothesis, Wilkin and colleagues devised three studies to assess physical activity levels of youth exposed to differing environmental influences (78). Activity was measured by accelerometer recordings continuously over 7 days. In the first, the physical activity levels of 307 young children (mean age 4.9 years) were compared between weekdays and weekends. In accordance with a central control of activity, average activity did not differ in the two periods. In the second study, levels of daily physical activity in older children (aged 7-11 years) were assessed in three schools with widely divergent hours of physical education (9.0, 2.2, and 1.8 hours per week). When in-school and out-of-school activities were combined, no differences were observed in total daily activity in the three schools. The third investigation revealed similar daily activity levels in children who lived in Glasgow and Plymouth, two cities in Great Britain of differing size, culture, and climate. The authors concluded that "together, the data reported here suggest that children of primary school age display consistency in the amount of physical activity they undertake, independently of opportunity, daily routine, background or culture. Such consistency raises the question of central control" (p. 1053).

Effects of Activity Interventions on Subsequent Physical Activity

Given the recognized importance of the issue, several research studies have investigated the effects of a programmed intervention of physical activity on subsequent levels of motor activity. These investigations, then, sought to identify the extent of *persistence* of augmented activity after an exercise program. Over the past decade, several reviews and meta-analyses have sought to consolidate findings into a general conclusion regarding the outcomes of these investigations performed in different population groups. For the most part, these reviews have consistently indicated a small but significant improvement in postintervention short-term activity levels, but the significance of such minor changes is uncertain.

Such analyses are confounded by the variety of study designs, variability of venues, and combination with dietary interventions. In addition, conclusions are often weakened by the common reliance on participant self-report rather than objective measures of physical activity as well as limited short-term follow-up. There are questions, too, about the influence of publication bias (journals are more likely to accept studies reporting positive rather than negative findings) and the fact that neither subjects nor investigators were blinded about the treatment groups or goals of participation in the study.

In 2008, van Sluijs and colleagues performed a literature search of published reports of physical activity levels after exercise interventions in subjects under 18 years of age that involved a nonprogram control group (75). They identified 33 studies in children and 24 in adolescents, among which they considered 42% to be of high scientific quality. Among all the studies, the great majority involved school-based interventions, and approximately half used parent or child report of activity level as the outcome marker. In the child studies, only a third used an objective measure of postprogram physical activity. In that group of reports, only 10 (18%) involved a follow-up period of at least 6 months.

Thirty-eight of the 57 studies (67%) described a positive effect of the exercise intervention on later levels of physical activity, a change that reached statistical significance in 27 of the studies (47%). Among the latter, increases in activity ranged from 2.6 minutes during physical education classes to a rise of 83 minutes per week of moderate to vigorous physical activity. Overall, about half of the participants became more active after the exercise program. Positive outcomes, however, were limited largely to the adolescent group, since the children demonstrated no or inconclusive changes in activity when the data were analyzed across different settings. The authors concluded, that "a lack of high quality evaluations hampers conclusions concerning effectiveness, especially among children" (75, p. 653).

Six years later, Biddle and colleagues performed a meta-analysis employing effect size to assess 22 studies of intervention outcomes in girls aged 5 to 11 years (7). (*Effect size* is a measure of the strength of an association in a practical sense and is independent of subject number. Usually calculated as the difference between the two mean population values for a variable divided by the pooled standard deviation, it provides insight into the extent that differences between two groups can be considered meaningful. Normally an effect size of 0.2 to 0.3 is considered small, 0.5 is moderate, and more than 0.8 is large.) The overall effect size in these reports of 0.31 was "small but significant," being equivalent to 12% greater physical activity for the subjects in the intervention group. It was concluded that "the small effect shown in the present meta-analysis suggests that behavior change may be challenging" (p. 128).

From the same research group, Pearson and others subsequently found similar findings of a small but significant effect in an analysis of studies assessing the effectiveness of interventions to increase physical activity among adolescent girls (48). The average treatment effect in this meta-analysis was 0.35 (95% confidence limits 0.12 to 0.58). These levels of effect size are consistent with those reported in a review of international activity intervention studies published between 2000 and 2011 by Heath and colleagues (30). The reported effect sizes in most were between 0.2 and 0.3.

Metcalf and others performed a review and meta-analysis of intervention outcomes in subjects under 16 years of age that differed by including only those studies in which (a) the intervention was at least 4 weeks in duration, (b) physical activity outcomes were objectively measured by accelerometry, and (c) outcomes were measured before or immediately after the intervention period (i.e., limited short-term effects) (47). The 30 investigations satisfying these criteria included 6,153 children, and articles were published between May 2003 and December 2011. Sixteen of the studies were considered to be of high methodological quality.

The analysis revealed a small but statistically significant effect of increase in both total activity and moderate or vigorous physical activity. The authors thought that "strong evidence exists from this analysis to suggest that physical activity interventions have a small to negligible effect on activity outcomes" (47). They estimated that the magnitude of the small improvements in activity identified in this review was equivalent to an addition of approximately 4 minutes more walking or running daily and that the clinical importance of such changes is likely to be minimal.

At the other end of the life span, Hobbs and colleagues reviewed 21 randomized controlled activity interventional studies involving adults aged 55 to 70 years (32). Of these, only 5 assessed activity by objective measures; the remainder relied on self-report of the participants. An average increase in activity outcomes was evident at the 12-month follow-up, with an increase equivalent to 2,197 pedometer steps per day. However, in the 8 studies that extended follow-up to 24 months, no sustained effect on physical activity levels was observed.

Chase and others reviewed the overall effectiveness of interventions to augment physical activity behavior in adults over 65 years (mean age 70 years) (17). The overall effect size for two-group posttest comparisons in 13,829 subjects was 0.18. This value was calculated to be equivalent to an increase of 620 steps per day.

Compensation in Response to Activity Interventions

If an activity-stat acts to stabilize overall activity energy expenditure as an isolated function, it would be expected that efforts to increase physical activity would be met, over time, by a compensatory fall in out-of-program exercise. Documenting the existence of such activity compensation would therefore serve as solid evidence for the activity-stat concept.

The initial studies that specifically addressed the question of activity compensation provided conflicting results. Dale and colleagues, for example, measured activity levels by accelerometers in 78 third- and fourth-grade children to determine if compensation for a school day of restricted activities would occur by increased activity in the after-school hours (21). The children wore monitors for two separate days when participation in recess and physical education class was eliminated and for another two days with 30 minutes of physical education and two outdoor recess periods. Total activity counts during the active school day were more than 10 times those of the restricted days. No compensatory increase in after-school activity was observed after the restricted day. Average activity levels (movement counts·min^{-1}) were 525 ± 306 and 246 ± 177 on active and restrictive days, respectively (figure 11.1).

This same research approach has been applied to animals as well. Lore reviewed 11 studies that measured physical activity in rats immediately after they had been confined for periods ranging from 5 hours to 8 days (42). Findings were mixed, with augmented activity described in some reports, while most revealed no changes.

Goran and Poehlman investigated the effect of an 8-week highly intense endurance exercise program on total energy expenditure in elderly adults aged 56 to 78 years (27). No changes were observed in total energy expen-

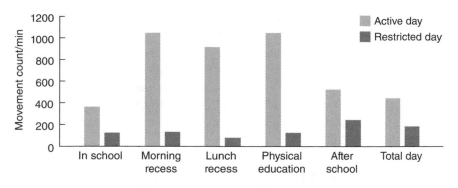

Figure 11.1   In the study of Dale and colleagues, average activity counts of physical activity were similar in days of active and restrictive activity, indicating no compensatory responses to exercise interventions.
Data from Corbin, Corbin, and Dale 2007.

diture, explained as a 62% reduction in activity energy expenditure outside the program.

Another study demonstrating compensatory changes in physical activity commensurate with the activity-stat hypothesis came from Ridgers and colleagues (56). Accelerometry data were used to examine whether 8- to 11-year-old children ($n = 248$) who were involved in more physical activity during a given day would be less active the following day and whether those who were sedentary would have increased activity on the subsequent day. They found that an additional 10 minutes of moderate to vigorous physical activity on any given day was associated with approximately 25 minutes less light-intensity activity and 5 minutes less moderate to vigorous activity the next day. Every additional 10 minutes involved in light activity was followed the next day by 4.6 minutes less light activity and 0.9 minutes less moderate to vigorous physical activity. And for every 10 minutes of sedentary time, the children spent 0.5 minute less sedentary time during the next day.

Shephard and colleagues reported that the addition of 5 hours per week of physical education by Canadian school children caused a small but statistically insignificant decline in weekday leisure activity (66). These authors concluded that "the possible existence of hypothalamic biofeedback mechanisms limiting total daily activity is discouraging for those planning physical education curricula. Nevertheless, our data suggest that any such effect is small" (p. 63).

Daily accelerometry movement counts were assessed by Goodman and others in 345 British children aged 8 to 13 years (25). On weekends and weekdays, an extra 1% of time in physical activity predicted a 0.21% to 0.60%

increase in proportion of the day spent in moderate to vigorous activity. No compensatory reductions in activity were observed.

Baggett and colleagues measured physical activity by accelerometry over 6 consecutive days in 6,918 eighth-grade girls from the Trial of Activity for Adolescent Girls Study (1). In this study, daily inactivity was observed to be negatively associated with total physical activity, causing the authors to conclude that their findings were "not consistent with the activitystat hypothesis" (p. 1193).

To further examine this issue, Gomersall and others provided an analysis of the research literature published as of the year 2014 of studies that examined compensatory changes in physical activity over time (24). Twenty-eight such reports were identified, only one of which was said to have specifically been designed to test the activity-stat hypothesis. Of these studies, approximately half (13 of them) described clear evidence of compensation and another 3 revealed mixed results (i.e., compensation is certain subgroups). The authors considered their analysis to indicate that "methodological approaches to testing compensation are mixed and support for the activitystat remains unclear" (p. 146).

Obviously, drawing any confident conclusion from these data regarding the existence of central control of physical activity that might function as an activity-stat is not possible. Reviews of studies regarding activity interventions from differing age groups consistently indicate a small mean improvement in outcome activity. But whether this has any clinical significance, and whether this speaks for or against central control of activity, is open to individual interpretation. These data are obfuscated by several critical factors, most particularly issues surrounding accuracy of measurement of physical activity outcomes (a minority of studies have employed objective measures), lack of long-term follow-up, and failure to consider interindividual variability.

Wilkin emphasized the weakness of studies demonstrating increases in activity in response measured for only a short duration after an activity intervention (77). "It is crucial," he noted, "to distinguish what may be short-term perturbation from long-term modulation" (p. 1274). He described an unpublished meta-analysis of studies involving 3,000 children in which activity outcomes were objectively measured. In this review, the largest effect sizes were observed in those investigations with the shortest duration, and an inverse relationship was observed between duration and outcome. This finding highlights the influence of long-term follow-up on results of activity interventions. Specifically, it demonstrates that the longer researchers wait after an activity intervention to conduct measurements, the less they observed the effect of that activity.

COMPENSATORY CHANGES IN CALORIC INTAKE

This response implies the existence of a master energy-stat that balances energy in and energy out to maintain a stable body weight and composition. (Recall that such a controller of energy balance does not necessarily imply a particular anatomic structure or even a system of neurological structures but rather one that, perhaps by biochemical mediators, would permit separate appetite and energy expenditure and other contributors of the energy balance equation to talk to each other.) In this scenario, the extra calories expended in the walking program would be compensated for by an equivalent amount of caloric intake through stimulation of appetite, resulting in a new steady state or set point but with unchanged body weight or composition. In this case, no compensatory decrease in physical activity would be expected after an exercise intervention, but dietary measurements should document an adaptive rise in food intake.

Thivel and colleagues acknowledged the intuitive nature of this response when they commented that "evidence suggests that energy expenditure and energy intake are actually closely inter-related, [and] it seems actually too simplistic to consider physical activity and food consumption as two independent ways to respectively manipulate EE and EI and thus control energy balance" (71, p. 59).

This response of the young patient would be in keeping with the general tenets of energy homeostasis and the role that control of physical activity might play in the global context of maintaining body weight, as outlined in the previous section. Such an adaptive outcome would be consistent, too, with an evolutionary-based mechanism by which the *milieu intérieur* is carefully maintained.

Those who are so convinced find it vexing, then, that experimental studies have largely failed to indicate compensatory responses of augmented caloric intake to physical activity interventions. These are reviewed in the previous section, but to recapitulate here, studies assessing energy intake after a period of physical activity intervention typically demonstrate no change in daily caloric intake, with a smaller percentage reporting equal frequency of increased or decreased food consumption (8, 9, 22, 35, 36). The great majority of such studies examined changes in caloric intake shortly after the exercise intervention (1-10 days), but the few medium-term (2-8 weeks) and long-term (2-12 months) studies revealed the same trends (8).

Blundell and King offered several explanations of why energy intake is only weakly coupled with activity energy expenditure (8). First, eating behavior is not governed simply by physiologic variables:

It is widely accepted that behavioral patterns can be held in place by environmental contingencies (relationships between cues and responses) by associations between physiological signals and salient environmental stimuli (including food stimuli), as well as by more obvious social and cultural influences. The major importance of this perspective is that, once established, a pattern of eating and food choice can be maintained independently of many physiological events. (p. S573)

Second, physical activities could alter postabsorptive physiological processes, such as alterations in energy efficiency or resting metabolic rate. However, such influences were considered by these authors to have only a weak influence on food intake eating behavior.

Third, it takes time, but eventually caloric intake will rise to compensate for the augmented activity energy expenditure. "This is clearly necessary," Blundell and King point out, "because the body could not tolerate a permanent energy balance or loss in body weight. Therefore, at some stage during the period of 'adjustment' some mechanism must 'kick in' to prevent a continuing energy deficit and further weight loss" (8, p. S577). According to this suggestion, such a compensation would create a new steady state or energy balance set point at a lower body weight than the original one (figure 11.2).

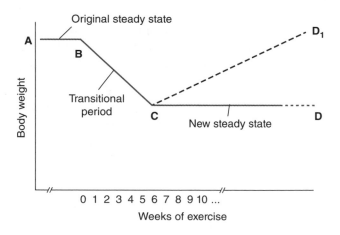

Figure 11.2   Proposed schema from Blundell and King indicating possible influence of delayed compensation after an activity intervention on body weight over time. From a steady state from A to B, exercise begins at B, causing a weight reduction to point C due to augmented energy expenditure. At point C, a delayed compensation of increased caloric intake is completed, causing a new set point to occur between C and D.

Reprinted, by permission, from J.E. Blundell and N.A. King, 1999, "Physical activity and regulation of food intake: Current evidence," *Medicine and Science in Sports and Exercise* 31(Suppl 11): S573-S583.

So, in this model, what will happen to the patient following the physician's exercise prescription? Over time (months?), his food intake would increase to compensate for the additional calories spent in walking. The unanswered question, though, is the duration that would be required for this adaptation. A rapid compensation in caloric intake might be expected to cause the energy balance set point to be unchanged, and the exercise intervention would have no effect on body weight. On the other hand, a delayed compensation that resulted in a period of energy imbalance might trigger a favorable resetting of the energy balance set point, with a fall in body weight. In other words, according to this model, *the efficacy of increased physical activity in affecting weight loss depends on the period over which compensatory adaptations in caloric intake occur.* This concept of regarding responses to perturbations of energy balance as a dynamic phenomenon, occurring over time, rather than a static one, is revisited in the discussion of obesity in chapter 12.

It is worth reiterating a critical point made several times in these discussions. The elephant in the room in all these questions of compensation is the matter of *time.* That is, compensatory adaptations of one part of the energy balance equation by another would not be expected to be instantaneous. But how long should it take? More specifically, how far out from an exercise intervention should an outcome measure of physical activity or appetite be measured to adequately capture (or not) a compensatory response? Days? Weeks? Months? The answer is currently unclear. A number of authors have weighed in on this issue:

• Hall and colleagues: "We are almost perpetually in energy imbalance on the time scale of hours or days. When a given day's intake and expenditure are plotted against each other, there is little association. It is only when they are averaged over much longer periods (weeks) that there begins to be a balance struck between intake and expenditure. This is a key point that is sometimes overlooked: energy balance as a concept depends on the time domain over which it is considered. We are always in energy imbalance, but the relative imbalance is greater over the short term than over the long term" (28, p. 991).

• Gomersall and colleagues: "If compensation [of physical activity] does occur, we are currently unsure of the time frame. It is unlikely that an activitystat would function within hours or a day and may be quite slow, operating not from day to day, but rather over weeks or even months" (24, p. 146).

• Blundell and colleagues: "There is growing evidence that it takes considerable time for EI [energy intake] to adjust to elevations of EE [energy expenditure]" (9, p. 655).

• Blundell and King: "The process of 'adjustment' is not immediate and may take several months" (8, p. S577).

This conclusion was also reflected in a Consensus Statement from the American Society for Nutrition:

Studies of short duration in which E_O [energy output] is increased by exercise showed no compensatory change in E_I [energy intake] over 1 or 2 d. As the duration of the studies increased, evidence for compensation emerged with longer-duration studies showing greater but incomplete compensation. (28, p. 991)

This factor of time poses some very real practical problems for those investigating energy balance and its perturbations in humans. As Hall and colleagues noted,

The characteristically long time scale (~1 y half-time) for human body weight and composition changes to occur make it difficult to study comprehensively the dynamics of energy balance because we cannot generally keep humans in metabolic wards for such extended periods. Even in free-living situations we cannot tract E_I or E_O for prolonged periods using current technologies. We are thus limited to "snapshots" of periods of ~2 wk. (28, p. 993)

It can be reasonably argued that when energy balance is perturbed, as with the patient who is walking to augment his caloric expenditure, such balance must be eventually reestablished. If not, he would be perpetually in negative caloric balance and would demonstrate an unabated loss of weight. The model set forth by Blundell of an adjustment period before caloric compensation occurs incorporates an adaptive resetting of the energy balance set point, which would not occur if the compensation period were short.

Here for the first time in these pages is a proposed means by which extrinsic environmental influences might serve to mold biologic control of activity. In the Blundell schema, a designed program of physical activity could lower the energy-stat set point as an outcome of delayed compensatory caloric intake, resulting in a loss of body weight.

In conclusion, it seems logical to place biologic regulation of physical activity into a general control of energy balance rather as an independent feedback mechanism. It should be expected, according to the principles surrounding maintenance of energy balance, that the patient in question should demonstrate augmented caloric intake in response to the walking program. The published literature indicates quite convincingly, however, that such short-term compensation does not often occur, an enigma that may be explained by a failure to appreciate the duration necessary for adaptive responses of increased energy intake to a rise in activity energy expenditure. Just how caloric intake by a given individual might compensate—fast or slow, complete or complete—for increases in physical activity might relate to other factors as well, including genetic influences and level of physical activity. Mayer and colleagues proposed, for instance, that regulation of body energy balance should be more precisely regulated when energy expenditure is high (45).

It may turn out that the element of time is more important than previously suspected. According to the Blundell model described previously (figure 11.2), a delay in compensation for increases in activity energy expenditure by a corresponding rise in caloric intake (the so-called transition period) is necessary for a downregulation of the energy steady state (the set point of the energy-stat model). If this occurs in the patient in the walking program, he will lose weight, which will be defended by the new set point against future perturbations. On the other hand, if compensation occurred over a short period, no alteration of the steady state would occur, and he would not lose weight while continuing to balance energy in and out by means of the original set point.

LONG-TERM CHANGES IN PHYSICAL ACTIVITY HABITS

This outcome speaks to a central preventive health strategy for promoting regular physical activity, particularly in the pediatric age group. Get children into the habit of regular exercise early on, it says, to create a foundation for a lifestyle of physical activity that will persist into adulthood, offering expected beneficial health outcomes. This approach, then, presupposes no threshold amount of health-promoting activity during childhood but instead makes the principal goal motivational methods that foster persistence. In this regard, the issue of determinism of physical activity levels turns from physiologic regulation of energy balance to a psychological one of behavior modification (60).

Does this really occur? How confident can a pediatrician be that young patients will carry forward their involvement in physical activity once an exercise prescription expires? A number of tracking studies have been performed to address this question, seeking to determine if individuals who are physically active at a young age remain so into the adult years. Obviously, such investigations are notoriously difficult to perform, given that activity assessments are required to be taken on the same people 20 to 30 years apart using the same measurement tools, and a large number of confounding variables need to be acknowledged that could alter activity habits (i.e., changes over this period in diet, participation in athletics, geography, health, and occupation).

In 2009, Telama published a review of 20 studies that provided physical activity tracking information in individuals from late childhood to the midadult years (70). None of these reports used objective means of measuring physical activity, relying instead on questionnaires, diaries, and family report. Average tracking coefficients (indicating the stability of activity over the duration of the study) were low: 0.24 (range 0.03 to 0.44) for studies of males and 0.25 (range 0.07 to 0.66) in females. Two of the studies in men and eight in the women revealed no statistically significant tracking of physical activity at all over the time period. At best, these studies appear to indicate a low to moderate tracking of physical activity levels from ages 9 to 16 years to ages 25 to 40 years. However, such investigations do not address the more critical issue here: Will an *increase* in a child's activity patterns through a physical activity intervention be expected to persist into the adult years? At present, then, there exists no experimental evidence one way or the other about the validity of this strategy concerning persistence of exercise habit.

Developmental psychologists have long been interested in the long-term outcomes of early childhood behavioral interventions, but most of their studies have surrounded the question of the influence of early education on subsequent cognitive abilities. However, in this research, they identify several possible mechanisms for instilling early habit formation that could have applicability to long-term persistence of physical activity behaviors. These include *conditioning*, the reinforcement of behaviors through external rewards (for activity, this would be pleasurable factors such as fun and social acceptance), and *imitation* (doing what others around you do, evidenced by language acquisition, smoking habits, and so on).

Particularly interesting is the phenomenon of *imprinting,* whereby stimuli applied to animals at a certain sensitive period early in life can create persistent behavioral patterns. Most commonly, such behaviors include social attachments, search-and-following behavior, and imitation of sexual activity. These kinds of behaviors, which occur without rewards or even any practical function, have traditionally been considered irreversible and neuronally fixed (43, 67).

Psychologists have long debated whether this imprinting occurs in human children and, if so, whether there are certain sensitive periods that would be most critical for their acquisition. Some say yes: "The conditional patterning, which in the animal is biologically inherited, is in the human species matched largely by socially transmitted forms, imprinting during what has long been known as the 'impressionable years'" (14, p. 97). Others argue no:

If the view is to be accepted that early exposure exercises a disproportionate influence on later development, the conclusion is inescapable that learning at this stage is particularly efficient and persistent. There is no evidence that this is the case, and [there is] a considerable amount of data which negates it. (18, p. 19)

Drawing on physiological mechanisms previously presented in this book, it is not difficult to implicate a role for biologic control in adaptation of long-term physical activity behaviors. For example, the process of imprinting may reflect epigenetic mechanisms that control gene expression, since "the pattern of expression of genes is determined by environmental levels of the organism in the context of its interaction with the environment" (43, p. 61). The extent to which a child's physical activity habits at age 10 might be fixed by early activity through genetic imprinting remains an intriguing though unexplored question. Still, such a concept is in keeping with current concepts of environmental influence on gene function.

Habit formation is based on intrinsic reward-seeking behavior. As described previously, certain dopaminergic neurons in the brain have been linked to the control of addictive forms of physical activity behavior in animal models, particularly compulsive wheel running in rodents. That intrinsic rewards from regular physical activity—be they psychological (self-image), social (acceptance by friends), or physical (attractiveness)—might drive the patient in question to persist in physical activities by such biologic systems is not incomprehensible.

To conclude, biologic control mechanisms that govern habitual activity might function beyond the realm of body energy balance. Motivation to sustain exercise may be linked to genetic effects and to reward systems within dopaminergic brain centers that are influenced by interventional strategies. Here, then, is another possible interface between biologic regulators and environmental determinants of physical activity.

IMPLICATIONS FOR HEALTH PROMOTION

From the standpoint of health promotion, which of the three possible responses to the intervention described in this chapter is preferable? The answer would seem to depend on the goal of the activity intervention. If the objective of the physician is to prevent obesity, to cause the patient to lose weight and decrease BMI, or at least not to witness a further rise in BMI, a delayed compensatory increase in caloric intake and a long-term change in activity level would be optimal. On the other hand, compensatory changes in other physical activity would render the physician's walking prescription useless, since any activity energy expenditure during the patient's walks would be compensated for by a reduction in other physical activities, resulting in no overall change in energy expenditure.

It's important to recognize, however, that salutary benefits of physical activity are not limited to weight control or energy balance. Many, in fact, are related to physical activity itself. As John Hay has stated:

> Not always is the concern with physical activity related to energy expenditure. It could be time spent weight bearing for bone development, time spent in social play for social development, time spent in solitary activity for psychological development, etc. Energy expenditure is a specific direct outcome obviously related to physical activity but is not always a necessary component to measure when physical activity is of interest. (29, p. 537)

The documented salutary outcomes from regular physical activity are multifold not only in number but also in possible mechanisms (73). Reduction in adrenal-sympathetic activity is probably responsible for lowering of blood pressure and diminished risk of ventricular tachyarrhythmias. Alterations in local prostaglandin synthesis may reduce cancer risk. Regular physical activity promotes physical fitness and improves functional capacity in the elderly. Stress loading on bones promotes bone density, retarding the course of osteoporosis in later adulthood. Improved lipid profile and antithrombosis contribute to diminished risk of coronary artery disease. Peripheral vascular endothelial function is improved by exercise training. Alterations in brain neurotransmitters (norepinephrine, dopamine, serotonin) and endogenous opioids (endorphins) are linked to the effects of regular exercise on mental health. Even in obese individuals, Shaibi and others have emphasized that, independent of weight loss, physical activity can favorably alter biomarkers of cardiovascular health (65). The mechanisms underlying these favorable effects of being physically active are not clearly understood, but they are obviously different and largely independent of energy balance.

Children do not generally suffer from coronary artery disease, strokes, osteoporosis, and peripheral vascular disease. Nonetheless, the clinical markers of these diseases in adults (such as myocardial infarction and cerebral vascular accidents) are recognized to be lifelong expressions of processes that begin during the childhood and adolescent years. Promotion of physical activity in youth is thus largely predicated on the concept of early amelioration of these pathologic processes that will result in adverse clinical outcomes in the adult years (59).

The point here is that improvements in physical activity itself, without concern regarding compensatory changes or maintenance of energy balance, can be expected to pay health dividends. By this reasoning, outcomes in response to a program of augmented exercise that involve net increases in physical activity may be salutary, regardless of influence on energy balance.

Even if the energy expenditure of a prescribed exercise program were offset by other changes in physical energy expenditure, the program would not be entirely without merit. The program would still be useful if the exercise intervention had a specific, unique goal, such as strength training in preparation for a football season or weight-bearing activities for an individual with a strong family history of early osteoporosis.

Understanding Obesity: The Biologic Perspective

Obesity—the abnormal accumulation of body fat—represents, by some means, a malfunction in the mechanisms by which energy balance is normally maintained. The laws of thermodynamics dictate such an indisputable conclusion. But what, exactly, has gone awry? The vast amount of research and interpretative discussion addressing this topic would extend far beyond the purview of this book. Still, given its intimate connection with biologic control (or not) of physical activity and other components of the energy balance equation, a brief excursion into the energy dynamics that result in excessive adiposity is warranted. What follows, then, is an overview of a biological approach to the etiology and, by extension, the prevention and treatment of obesity. Although admittedly superficial, it does capture the essence of the issues confronting those endeavoring to combat this growing menace to health worldwide. In addition, it becomes apparent that unraveling the processes underpinning the deranged control of energy balance that results in obesity may provide insights into the essential nature of how such regulation normally functions.

FIRST LAW OF THERMODYNAMICS

Considerations of the etiology of obesity need to be placed in the context of the first law of thermodynamics. In the mid-1800s, the work of at least 10 European scientists, mainly Rudolf Clausius in Germany and William Thomson in Great Britain, led to the formulation of the first law of thermodynamics: *Energy can be transformed from one form to another but cannot be created or destroyed* (20). The human machine is a metabolic one, converting chemical energy in from the diet to physiologic function as energy out, and the dynamic flux involved in such balance must conform to this thermodynamic principle. Any excess in energy intake versus energy output, or vice versa, must be accounted for by alterations in energy stored in the body. That is, the rate of change in body energy stores is equal to the difference between the rates of energy intake (dietary calories consumed) and energy output (principally basal metabolic rate, physical activity, and thermic effect of food) (28). Homeostatic mechanisms normally maintain tight control of energy balance to stabilize body weight as an evolutionary-driven survival mechanism. As a consequence, body weight in adults is normally remarkably constant over time.

OBESITY AS AN ERROR IN ENERGY BALANCE

The obese state is an outcome of an error in the regulation of body energy balance. The mismatch between caloric intake and energy expenditure that results in excess storage of body fat is a very small one. Schoeller calculated that a 10 kg excessive gain in weight accumulated over a period of 10 years would result from an average daily imbalance of just 20 kcal per day (64). This observation has given rise to the popular notion that becoming obese is a matter of consuming only a single extra potato chip each day (6). Fortunately for lovers of potato chips, higher energy gaps leading to obesity have been reported. For instance, in the longitudinal Kiel Obesity Prevention Study, the 90th percentile of energy gap in normal-weight children 1 to 14 years old who became obese 4 years later was 53 to 72 kcal per day (49). (The energy content of an average potato chip is about 7 kcal.) Such information has been used to point out that even very small changes in daily energy expenditure sustained over extended time should be expected to be effective in obesity management strategies.

Some researchers have considered the driving factor responsible for the energy balance mismatch leading to obesity to occur on the caloric intake side of the ledger (6, 23). Finelli and colleagues, for example, commented:

> There is at the present time little evidence for major adaptations of energy expenditure during overfeeding, and changes in body weight and composition appear to be the major factors that, by increasing energy expenditure, allow energy balance to be restored. The body weight gain may therefore be seen as an adaptative change to overfeeding. (23, p. 1)

Others would disagree, claiming that maladaptive changes on the out side of the energy equation are culpable in the balance mismatch causing obesity.

It should be remembered, too, that the major contributors on both sides of the energy balance equation (caloric intake, BMR, activity energy expenditure, TEF) demonstrate a progressive decline in values (in respect to body size) over time, particularly dramatic during the childhood years. Establishment of energy balance, then, must be viewed as a dynamic process. It is possible, then, that the failure of a central controller to equate energy in and out in the development of obesity reflects an error in matching the *rates of change* of these variables as an individual ages (58).

BEHAVIORAL EXPLANATIONS FOR ENERGY IMBALANCE

The error in the mechanism of energy balance has traditionally been considered to reflect behavioral changes in response to environmental factors. If hundreds of thousands of years of evolutionary pressures have fashioned a genetically based means of stabilizing body weight, how can one explain the dramatic population-wide rise in obesity in the brief span of the last 50 years? The short duration and pervasive nature of this trend are too short to be explained by genetic mutation. Instead, the general consensus holds that the current rise in obesity reflects the combined effects in advanced societies of easy access to high-calorie, inexpensive foods in conjunction with the technological advances that have virtually eliminated the need for strenuous physical activity in daily living. The behavioral responses of the individual to these contemporary advances of human civilization, so the concept goes, involve excessive food consumption and the adaptation of a sedentary lifestyle, resulting in the energy imbalance that results in excessive accumulation of body fat.

The failure of the evolutionary-designed energy balance control system to react to this surfeit of caloric intake has been explained by the one-sided protective nature of this balancing mechanism. The evolutionary pressure in the distant past served to prevent body weight loss at a time when food availability was typically limited. A negative caloric balance was the survival risk. There existed no evolutionary pressure to avoid a positive balance of energy, since this rarely, if ever, occurred. Weight loss, not weight gain, was the survival issue. As Berthoud emphasized:

> Given the harsh environmental conditions that characterized the life of a majority of our human ancestors, those most likely to reach reproductive age must have had a regulatory system that was efficient in procuring and metabolizing energy. Such "thrifty" genes that were selected are involved in many aspects of the regulatory system, from

discerning perception of nutrients in the environment to an efficient transformation of calories into muscle work and body heat. . . . [But] genes that worked perfectly well in the nutritionally restrictive environment of our ancestors are now challenged with an abundance of food and lack of physical activity. (6, pp. 486-487)

Not all are in agreement with this explanation. In an article titled "Ten Putative Contributors to the Obesity Epidemic," McAllister and 22 coauthors suggested that a "myopic emphasis on the 'big two' [food intake and physical activity] has caused the popular media, and perhaps some researchers as well, to neglect the potential contributions of other factors to the balance between energy intake and expenditure" (46, p. 869). They outlined evidence to support other potential contributors to the development of obesity, including infection by microorganisms, inflammation, endocrine disorders, greater fecundity of obese individuals, and drug effects.

GENETIC EXPLANATIONS FOR ENERGY IMBALANCE

If the model of environmental-induced effects on eating and activity behaviors were solely responsible for the energy imbalance that causes obesity, everyone in the population would be obese. But everyone in the population, confronting the same environmental pressures, is not obese. Thus, individual differences in susceptibility to the obesogenic influences of contemporary societies must exist on a genetic level.

Twin studies have indicated a 40% to 70% heritability influence on common obesity (that not associated with particular disease states or syndromes). Given the accepted notion, then, of genetic-induced susceptibility for excess adiposity among individuals, an extensive research effort has been undertaken to identify the specific genes involved. These investigations have been facilitated by the many creative investigative techniques now available to molecular geneticists, including genome-wide linkage studies, candidate gene analysis, and genome-wide association studies (see refs. 31 and 74 for reviews). Not unexpectedly, perhaps, the genes-for-obesity picture has developed as more complex than one might have hoped. As of 2012, more than 50 genetic variants have been identified that are linked to obesity and distribution of fat (74). These genes involve the regulation of energy balance, appetite, lipid metabolism, and adipogenesis. Taken collectively, however, these do not account for the entire hereditary influence of factors leading to excessive fat accumulation.

It is suspected that epigenetic mechanisms may play a prominent role in the heritability of obesity. These, it will be recalled from an earlier discussion, involve agents that regulate the expression of genes without altering their basic DNA structure. These epigenetic factors often act by the process of DNA methylation and histone modifications that select certain gene information for outcome actions. The particular importance of this function is that such epigenetic modifiers (a) can be influenced by environmental factors and (b) in some cases may be transmittable from parent to child through the sexual gametes (3). Imprinted genes have been recognized that influence tissue differentiation, development, and metabolic functions. Evidence also exists that epigenetic factors operating during critical periods in early childhood development may increase risk of obesity (76).

In their review of this topic, Herrera and others concluded that "the epigenetic contributions to common forms of obesity are still largely unknown but from rare syndromes and animal models we conclude that it is likely that both genetic and environmental effects on epigenetics will in turn be associated with obesity" (p. 44). They continue,

> Despite the success of [new genetic techniques] in obesity loci identification, we still explain a low fraction of the inter-individual variation of obesity. Extensive work including identification of more obesity susceptibility loci, a better understanding of the gene(s) through which the effect is executed, as well as further molecular and physiological characterization of the associated genes, is now necessary before any of these findings will lead to any useful therapeutic interventions. (31, p. 44)

Several mechanisms exist by which genetic information would act to create vulnerability to obesity. One's complement of genetic material and its expression as regulated by epigenetic mechanisms could be manifest in physiologic alterations that lead to the obese state.

Metabolic Processes

One of the first ideas presented to explain obesity was that obese individuals had unique differences in the metabolic processes that contribute to energy expenditure. Specifically, it was thought that in obese people, these components of the out side of the energy equation were somehow more efficient—requiring less energy—than in the nonobese. This intuitively sensible concept has triggered a voluminous amount of research aimed at identifying the specific processes that might be involved. The data are mixed, and no definite metabolic weakness has been identified that could clearly account for such disadvantages for the obese.

A number of studies have been performed with Pima Indians, who have a particular unexplained predilection for obesity. These have indicated that a low resting metabolic rate and higher respiratory quotient (a measure of the relative amount of energy derived from fat and carbohydrate) are associated with long-term weight gain (53, 81). Using these data, and assuming that two-thirds of variability in body fat content is established by genetic factors, Ravussin and Bogardus estimated that of this genetic influence, 12% could be accounted for by resting metabolic rate, 5% by respiratory quotient, and 10% by spontaneous physical activity (52). The remaining 40% was presumed to reflect other factors, including food intake.

Speed of Response to Imbalance

Body energy balance is often considered as maintaining a static equilibrium, matching caloric intake against those factors that determine energy expenditure. Indeed, this balance is often depicted figuratively in publications as a scale with energy intake on one pan and energy output on the other. In fact, however, maintenance of energy balance is a dynamic function, and the matching of caloric intake and energy expenditure needs to be viewed as occurring over time (figure 12.1).

The concept that individual variability in rate of compensation for a perturbation of energy balance could influence subsequent outcomes in terms of weight gain is introduced in chapter 9. As outlined by Blundell and King (8), the magnitude of weight loss expected from the excess caloric expenditure of a physical activity intervention could depend on the rapidity as well as the completeness with which a compensatory augmentation in food intake could occur.

The same phenomenon can be described in terms of an obesogenic mechanism. Suppose a young man, previously lean and in perfect energy balance, finds employment in a doughnut shop. Seduced by the surrounding pastries, he finds that his caloric intake quickly jumps by 400 calories per day. What will be the effect on his body weight? Four million years of evolutionary pressure has equipped this young man with a central mechanism that demands a matching of this excessive energy intake with a caloric-equivalent energy expenditure through increases in RMR or TEF, or through voluntary or involuntary physical activity. If such an adaptive compensation were rapid, no change would be expected in his body weight—he would quickly be back in energy balance. But if the compensation were delayed by weeks or months, weight gain would occur during this adaptation, since this is a period in which energy intake exceeds energy expenditure. When compensation is finally achieved, his energy balance mechanism would be operating at a new set point at the greater weight as the steady state. (Of course, if he continues to indulge, further weight gain would be expected.) By this scenario, then, people genetically

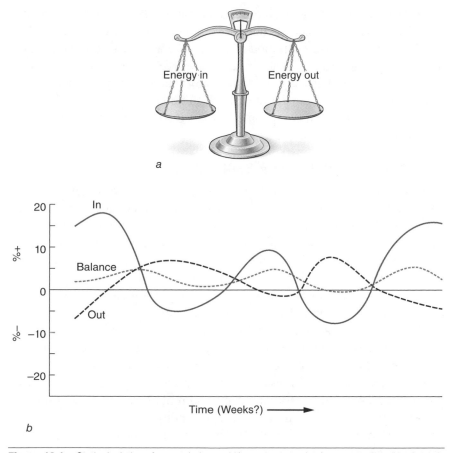

Figure 12.1   Static depiction of energy balance *(a)* is more appropriately presented as *(b)* a dynamic fluctuation of energy in and energy out over time.

predisposed to slow compensation would be more vulnerable to obesity, fast responders less so.

This concept has been supported by the neuroimaging study of Matsuda and colleagues (44). These investigators compared the effects of glucose ingestion on hypothalamic function by functional magnetic resonance imaging (fMRI, a noninvasive imaging method that estimates regional metabolic activity in the brain) in 10 obese men and 10 lean men. After glucose ingestion, inhibitory signals were observed in the paraventricular and ventromedial nuclei in the lean subjects that were significantly delayed in the obese (6.4 ± 0.5 versus 9.4 ± 0.5 min, respectively).

Other data indicate that a considerable interindividual variability is observed in the magnitude of responses to perturbations of energy balance.

For example, King and others measured change in BMR ranging from −230 calories to +320 calories and change in body weight from −12 kg to +1 kg in subjects after a 12-week period of supervised aerobic training on a fixed diet (36) (see figure 9.6 in chapter 9). This degree of variability in the magnitude and temporal aspects of compensatory adaptations may account for individual susceptibility to obesity as well as explain the marked differences commonly observed among people in their response to obesity treatment interventions of diet and exercise (36).

Deranged Biochemical Messengers

As previously described, several biochemical mediators contribute to energy balance, ranging from agents in the gastrointestinal tract that monitor volume of food intake to the central nervous system neurotransmitter system responsible for integrating homeostatic information. Impaired function of any of these messengers—controlled by genetic directives—could be responsible for disturbing energy balance leading to the obese state.

Leptin, a well-established metabolic messenger governed by genetic control, acts differently in individuals who are obese. Fat people exhibit high levels of circulating leptin, which demonstrate little change when this agent is administered exogenously. From this observation, it can be assumed that the obese are in a state of leptin resistance (6). Why this should be is not known. The same picture of leptin resistance is observed in seasonal animals, who during hibernation are sensitive to leptin administration when leptin levels are normally low yet show little response to leptin in the summer when levels are high. Leptin function is controlled by hypothalamic neuronal signaling, leading some to suggest that reversible leptin resistance is a normal physiological neuronal function in seasonal animals (38).

Of course, such observational descriptions of leptin function in overweight humans provide no insights regarding the direction of the cause-and-effect arrow. Whether alterations in leptin might be a causative factor of obesity or, instead, an outcome of the obese state is not at all clear. As the following chapter notes, the concept that alteration of biochemical messengers might influence energy balance provides a potential mechanism for pharmacologic treatment of obesity.

IMPLICATIONS FOR TREATMENT AND PREVENTION

The scenario outlined previously permits a conclusion that, as previously emphasized by many authors, obesity can be viewed as a model example of the interaction of genetics and environment. More specifically, it can be suggested from this thought process that three central factors are most likely responsible for the growing problem of obesity:

- *Environmental*: sociocultural and technological changes in availability of inexpensive, high-calorie foods coupled with declining necessity for physical activity in daily living
- *Behavioral responses* to this obesogenic milieu: excessive food consumption and sedentary lifestyle
- *Biological mechanisms* that underlie energy imbalance: genetic-based susceptibility, reflected as maladaptive alterations in metabolic processes, compensatory adaptations, and biochemical signalers that normally serve to maintain energy balance

From this construct, one can suggest priorities for health-based interventions with the objective of preventing and treating obesity. Altering the environmental milieu, the proposed basic factor underlying the rise in obesity, would be optimal; however, to face it realistically, this is unlikely to be successful on any large scale. As Bouchard and Blair commented,

It will be a daunting task to change the course of nations that have progressively become quite comfortable with an effortless lifestyle in which individual consumption is almost unlimited. . . . [Some] have argued that the increase in the prevalence of overweight and obesity appears to be unstoppable as a side effect of modernization. (12, p. S500)

However, most efforts to date have focused on altering behavior through education, environmental manipulation, structured programs, promotion of physical education, involvement of physicians, and so forth. Although recent evidence exists that the rise of obesity has abated somewhat, such interventions have not demonstrated any dramatic long-term success despite several decades of intensive public health efforts. Perhaps this could be explained by the stubborn nature of evolutionary-directed energy set points in resisting the negative energy balance necessary for losing weight.

Ultimately, it may be best to view obesity as a biological disturbance rather than a behavioral one. Efforts to understand the physiologic underpinnings of energy balance may in the long run provide the best chance to alter the environmental–behavioral aspects of the obesity epidemic that are resistant to change. Gene therapy, treatment with transcription agents with epigenetic potential, identification of people at genetic risk, pharmacologic agents, factors that could alter the energy set point—these are all approaches that could provide a means of normalizing physiological responses to threats of energy imbalance. Some of these are addressed in chapter 13. Clearly, to achieve this goal, a great deal more needs to be done in order to understand the nature of the physiological disturbances in the obese state.

However, not all experts have seen it this way. For example, Zheng and colleagues argued the following:

> Common obesity results when individual predisposition to deal with a restrictive environment as engraved by genetics, epigenetics, and/or early life experience, is confronted with an environment of plenty. Therefore, increased adiposity in prone individuals should be seen as a normal physiological response to a changed environment, not in pathology of the regulatory system. The first line of defense should ideally lie in modifications to the environment and lifestyle. (80, p. S8)

Altering the Biologic Control of Activity

I n 2002, Sue Kimm and colleagues published particularly salient longitudinal data from the National Heart, Lung, and Blood Institute Growth
and Health Study on the trends in physical activity of adolescent girls
(34). In this study, a total of 1,213 black girls and 1,166 white girls from
urban regions were followed annually from the ages of 9 or 10 years until
18 or 19 years. Leisure-time physical activity was assessed with a validated
questionnaire, and using reported activities and their frequencies, equivalent
MET scores (per week) were calculated.

A progressive fall in activity was observed in both groups, describing a
curve not unlike that observed in the general population of adolescents (as
well as animals) noted in chapter 2 of this book. Over the 10 years of the
study, the average activity score fell from an initial 27.3 to 0 in the black
subjects and from 30.8 to 11.0 in the white subjects. When they were 16 to
17 years old, no habitual leisure-time activity was reported by 56% and 31%
of the black and white subjects, respectively. In analyzing these trends, four
factors were found to contribute to the rate of decline of activity in these girls:
lower level of parent education, cigarette smoking (white girls), pregnancy
(black girls), and greater adiposity (by body mass index).

A number of pertinent lessons can be drawn from this report. To start
with, it conforms to other data indicating that the level of physical activity
declines significantly during the early years of life as a normal biological
phenomenon. This study is a model of how assessment of factors that could
modify activity habits should be designed. Snapshots of determinant variables influencing short-term activity outcomes to weeks-long intervention
programs provide little insights. More important is how such interventions

might modify the downward trend expected in activity during an extended period.

This is one of very few investigations that have addressed a critical issue here: Is it possible that extrinsic factors can favorably bend upward the normally descending curve of activity levels in adolescents? In fact, the findings indicate that such an effect is likely—in this case, in respect to socioeconomic factors, smoking, and pregnancy—which provokes some very concrete therapeutic considerations:

> Some of the identified risk factors for declining activity could be helpful in prioritizing resources to reach more vulnerable girls. Moreover, some determinants of declining activity levels, such as teenage pregnancy and cigarette smoking, are possible targets of structured interventions to increase physical activity among adolescents. (34, p. 714)

This study, then, provides direct evidence that both biological regulation of physical activity (as manifest by the progressive decline in activity with age) and manipulation of environmental factors can influence activity habits. The following sections reinforce this concept with information indicating that biologic control may be altered by extrinsic influences as well as by personal will and hedonistic behavior. At present, the relative importance of intrinsic versus such extrinsic influences on motor behavior remains a central but unanswered question.

PLASTICITY OF BIOLOGIC SET POINTS

Biologic regulators that govern body physiologic functions are products of millions of years of evolutionary pressure. They should not, intuitively, be expected to be readily modifiable over time by extrinsic perturbations. However, clear examples of such shifts of homeostatic set points in response to environmental factors do exist.

Body temperature is normally tightly controlled by hypothalamic regulators to within a degree of 98.6 °F (37 °C) in respect for demands of thermal constancy of metabolic functions. Yet release of pyrogens in the bloodstream in response to infection and inflammation triggers the actions of prostaglandins in the brain, which shift the body temperature set point upward by as much as 4 °F (~2 °C). The resulting fever is considered to aid the body's immune system in combating the invading organisms. Antipyretics, drugs that are used to treat fever, such as aspirin, act by lowering prostaglandin levels, thereby bringing about a drop in the temperature set point.

As noted previously, all homeostatic set points in the body vary in a diurnal pattern. These circadian rhythms are intrinsic, with a periodicity of just over

24 hours. The pattern of these shifts in set points is altered, or *entrained,* by environmental influences, particularly light–dark cycles, which reset the rhythm periodicity to 24 hours. In this example, then, the level of biologic set points is affected by both intrinsic and extrinsic factors.

In the discussions in this book, it has been obvious that in the development of obesity, energy set points become readjusted to higher levels in response to a positive energy balance; that is, "obesity itself can often be viewed as a condition of body energy regulation at an elevated set point" (33, p. 1882S). A similar shift of set point may occur in control of blood pressure in individuals with hypertension, in whom physiologic regulators are adjusted to establish a steady state at higher levels.

Hibernation by animals is a classic example of biologic set points being not only modified but essentially eliminated altogether (69). During such periods, the metabolic rate of a bat has been reported to be 1% to 4% of that in the normal resting condition. At the same time, *homeothermy*—maintenance of body temperature—is virtually abandoned, with body temperature falling to close to 0 °C.

These examples illustrate that supposedly deterministic biologic controllers are not necessarily immutable. Such observations imply that efforts to improve the physical activity habits of the population by manipulating environmental factors might be successful even in the presence of a central nervous system controller of physical activity.

CAN COGNITIVE WILL OVERRIDE BIOLOGIC CONTROL?

The answer to this question is unclear. Reasonable arguments and examples can, in fact, be mounted on both sides of the issue. For example, a clear explanation for why animals, including humans, need to periodically sleep has not been forthcoming. Some restorative function, particularly neurological, has been supposed. For whatever reason sleep is required, the need to sleep cannot be overcome by cognitive decision making and will. In experiments of acute sleep deprivation, volunteers begin to complain of depression, confusion, memory loss, hallucinations, headaches, and decline in cognitive function as early as 48 hours without sleep, and sustained periods of sleeplessness become intolerable (13). With prolonged sleep deprivation, the brain will begin to shut down and automatically initiate periods of brief unconsciousness called microsleep (51). Long-term sleep deprivation over 2 to 3 weeks will cause death in laboratory animals (54). As much as one might wish, then, it is not possible by a person's will to avoid the biologic imperative of sleep. Similar nonperturbable functions are equally obvious, such as one encountered in attempting to hold one's breath.

Still, it is possible to override the control of food intake through personal decision. Defenders of noble purposes have starved themselves to death by hunger strikes. Even body fluid balance, normally carefully maintained by hormonal and renal homeostatic mechanisms, may be overturned by voluntary overdrinking of water, leading to life-threatening hyponatremia during marathon running (57). Athletes performing in high environmental temperatures may will themselves to persevere in the face of elevations in body temperature that threaten heatstroke and even death, even assuming a central brain governor whose goal is to limit exercise in the name of safety from such adverse outcomes (61). These examples illustrate that in certain situations, cognitive influences can override well-recognized biologic controllers.

CAN HEDONISTIC BEHAVIOR OVERRIDE BIOLOGIC CONTROL?

A common argument against the function of a biologic regulator of activity energy expenditure holds that human beings, unlike animals, are equipped with the cognitive facility to decide whether or not to exercise (6, 11). This capacity, then, to actively engage voluntarily in pleasurable, motivated activities (like playing a game of basketball, dancing until dawn in a nightclub, taking a bicycle trip in the country), termed *hedonistic* activities, might be expected to override any unconscious controller of physical activity. The same pleasure-seeking drive leads to overindulgence in food. The evidence lies, according to this argument, in the current obesity epidemic and the effect of hedonistic behavior in the milieu of the comforts of a technological society.

The counterargument is that the seemingly voluntary nature of eating and scheduled activities remains, despite all appearances, part of an overall energy balance scheme that is regulated by intrinsic control. Over time, the energy expended in such purposeful activities will be compensated for in the name of a balanced energy equation. This is evidenced by the observations that body weight is largely stable in the course of major voluntary caloric expenditures, such as heavy labor (45), training for a marathon (50), and competing in the Tour de France (63). Yes, this argument goes, activities such as willfully participating in physical activities and partaking of a large Thanksgiving meal do override a healthy biologic controller, but only temporarily. Given time, the biologic control of both activity and energy balance prevails. The basic problem underlying the development of obesity is not behavioral but biological, a faulty control mechanism leading to minor imbalances of energy in and out and to subsequent accumulation of body fat.

Which of these camps is in the right is currently unresolved. Perhaps it is likely that the true mechanisms underlying energy balance and the development of obesity will be found to rest in some combination of the two viewpoints.

Borer contended that "our understanding of the regulation of energy balance is impeded by preoccupation with a homeostatic view of this mechanism and comparative inattention to non-homeostatic motivational and physiological processes controlling feeding, spontaneous physical activity, and metabolism" (11, p. 114). She outlined lines of evidence that were considered inconsistent with a homeostatic function of feeding and spontaneous activity, including that (a) caloric consumption is strongly affected by factors such as food availability, social context, portion size, and palatability; (b) with increased food consumption, the extent of rapid gains in weight and body fat do not reflect homeostatic regulation; and (c) a dose-dependent rise in negative hormonal feedback is not observed as body fatness increases in response to excessive caloric intake.

Experimental evidence exists to support mechanisms by which hedonist behavior might trump the energy balance system. For instance, leptin is active by receptors not only in the hypothalamus but also in regions of the brain associated with pleasure and reward-stimulated behavior (e.g., hippocampus, neocortex, thalamus, caudal brain stem). The question is, then, in a time of high food availability, why does leptin not inhibit these hedonistic centers as it should also do for homeostatic hypothalamic control (6)? As noted previously, in humans, it fails to do so by assumed leptin resistance, as evidenced by high leptin levels.

Even more to the point, neurological connections have been observed between the hypothalamus and cortical regions of the brain involved in motivational aspects toward pleasurable eating and activity behavior. Based on such findings, Berthoud proposed that "accumbens-hypothalamus projections might engage the hypothalamic peptidergic systems known to be involved in homeostatic appetite control and that this might be an important pathway for the 'cognitive' and 'emotional' brain to override homeostatic regulation" (6, p. 494). On the other hand, it might be equally argued that the arrow of physiological function goes in the opposite direction, that such connections between involuntary homeostatic and voluntary cognitive centers might be a means by which the former incorporates the latter in the overall scheme of energy balance.

Perhaps a reasonable conciliatory viewpoint of this conflict is best expressed in the words of Zheng and others:

Thus the traditional view of neural circuits regulating energy homeostasis has been expanded to include neural mechanisms of learning and memory, reward, attention, decision-making, mood, and emotionality. Adequate supply of energy is simply too important as not to include these powerful neural processes. To distinguish eating driven by internal, metabolic hunger signals in the absence of metabolic need, the terms "homeostatic" and "non-homeostatic" controls of appetite have recently been adopted. In light of the intimate neural interactions between these two classes of signals, this distinction may have been premature. Metabolic signals can modulate the cortico-limbic systems involved in higher brain functions, and the cortico-limbic systems can hijack the behavioral/metabolic effector mechanisms controlling energy balance. Together they serve one purpose—to maintain an optimal internal milieu in harmony with the external world. (80, p. S11)

These arguments focus on hedonistic (pleasure-seeking) behavior supplanting biologic control of food intake, which, as noted previously, have been extended to contentions that similar behaviors might underlie hedonistic drives for physical activity. Experimental evidence does not currently exist to support or refute this argument.

ROLE OF SPONTANEOUS PHYSICAL ACTIVITY AND NEAT

Spontaneous physical activity (SPA) is generally considered as all forms of activity energy expenditure that do not involve planned voluntary physical activity that is engaged in for health or pleasure (i.e., sports). Nonexercise activity thermogenesis (NEAT) is defined as the energy expenditure involved in SPA. Some uncertainty exists regarding just which activities are included in SPA. Levine and Kotz defined NEAT as including "all those activities [besides volitional sporting-like exercise] that render us vibrant, unique, and independent beings such as going to work, playing guitar, toe-tapping and dancing" (40, p. 310). Others have considered SPA and NEAT from a more restrictive view as activities that one doesn't think about, such as energy expenditure from posture, fidgeting, holding a book, moving about the house, and climbing stairs.

Energy spent through NEAT varies markedly not only among individuals but within the same person from day to day. Its contribution to total daily energy expenditure can vary from 15% to over 50% (39).

Research evidence indicates that NEAT responds to states of energy imbalance. When Levine and colleagues overfed adult volunteers by 1,000 calories per day over 8 weeks, 531 calories were expended through increased energy expenditure and 432 calories were stored (41). Voluntary exercise was stringently maintained at constant low levels. Increases in BMR and TEF increased by an average of 79 and 137 calories, respectively, meaning that 328 kcal or 62% of the rise in total energy expenditure response to overfeeding was caused by increases in NEAT. In this study, the changes in NEAT directly predicted the resistance to fat gain. Similar responses of fall in NEAT have been reported with negative energy balance (39).

It might be assumed that factors influencing spontaneous activity in animals are similar to those affecting NEAT in humans (i.e., both reflecting involuntary, noncognitive energy expenditure) (15). If so, the supporting data for homeostatic systems and neurochemical mediators for energy in control in animals outlined in early chapters of this book could be manifest as NEAT in humans. Leptin and orexin, for example, have been considered as prime candidates for controlling NEAT (40). There is no current proof for this in human beings. In fact, certain activities in rodents, such as wheel running, have been considered analogous not to NEAT in humans but rather to hedonistic, pleasure-seeking behaviors.

PHARMACOLOGICAL MANIPULATION OF PHYSICAL ACTIVITY REGULATORS

Thorburn and Proietto, recognizing the many chemical agents known to alter activity energy expenditure, suggested that biological control mechanisms for regulating physical activity might be modified by pharmacological interventions as a means of treating obesity (72). Currently, several drugs have been approved for obesity management, such as phentermine-topiramate, Orlistat, and naltrexone-bupropion, but these all act by diminishing the caloric intake side of energy balance by either reducing gastrointestinal fat absorption or suppressing appetite. In adults, these medications add 3% to 9% weight loss compared to placebo when combined with traditional obesity interventions (diet, exercise) (78).

Keesey and Hirvonen provided evidence to suggest that anorectic drugs may also bring about changes in body weight, partially by altering the set point for energy regulation (33). They note,

> Anorectic drugs . . . are effective in suppressing food intake only until body weight declines to a particular level. Intake then returns to essentially normal, although body weight remains at a reduced level. Traditionally, tolerance to the anorectic agent has been offered as the explanation for the drug's failure to continue suppressing food intake.

However, an alternative explanation is that anorectic drugs produce their effects by lowering the body weight set point. (p. 1881S)

The efforts to identify such drugs have taken advantage of recent research insights into the neurobiology of appetite, including pharmaceuticals that might affect dopamine function, as well as the anorexigenic actions of opioid antagonists and serotonin on the hypothalamus (2). For example, the deletion of two negative regulators of leptin action (suppressor of cytokine signaling or tyrosine phosphate PTB1B) has been found to protect rodents from developing leptin resistance and subsequent obesity (6).

At present no drugs are available for obesity management that specifically augment activity energy expenditure. Yet the knowledge that biochemical mediators, such as leptin and the melanocortin system, govern activity energy expenditure (reviewed earlier in this book) clearly suggests the potential for a similar research focus on pharmacologic agents to augment physical activity. As Ceccarini and others concluded,

In light of the recent difficulties in finding drugs with a safe and durable impact on body weight, an alternative approach to be employed in the future may be represented by stimulating physical activity and leptin sensitivity or reproducing its beneficial effect on weight control. Iden- tification of gene variants positively associated with beneficial effects of increased locomotor activity in obese individuals may further help in the selection of subsets of patients potentially responding to such therapeutic approach. (16, p. 129)

Castañeda and colleagues have suggested that future pharmaceutical inter- ventions to stimulate spontaneous physical activity may be most effective in treating obesity since these forms of activity have the greatest variability of all the contributors to energy expenditure (15). There also exists the future prospect of identifying specific epigenetic transcription factors that favorably modify gene action for activity and weight reduction.

Because of concern over side effects, anorectic drugs have been used only with caution for treatment of obesity in the pediatric age group. At the time of this writing, only a single agent, orlistat, has FDA approval in this age group (10). Drug treatment for behavior-related diseases in youth has often been considered an anathema; for example, much objection has been raised to the use of methylphenidate for children with hyperactivity disorders. At the same time, none would object to employing drugs in life-threatening conditions, such as malignancies or serious infections. It can be argued that grossly obese youth are threatened with a not-dissimilar threat to health, and the development of pharmaceutical approaches that would aid weight loss through increased physical activity might be a more optimal approach than surgery and attempts at behavior modification.

The identification of drugs that favorably alter biologic regulation of activity energy expenditure might bear utility not just for those with obesity. Such agents have already been identified that promote motor recovery in patients after cerebral vascular accidents (4). Enrichment of motor behavior and upregulation of trophic factors in the central nervous system have been considered important in treating patients recovering from brain injuries (37) and Parkinson's disease (68).

Epilogue

To summarize, the evidence in both animals and humans is persuasive that a biologic controller participates in the regulation of habitual physical activity. The diverse sources of this evidence presented in part I are particularly impressive. Levels of activity decline over the life span in both human beings and animals. Activity differences between males and females appear to have a biological basis as well as the assumed sociocultural influence. Physiologic factors relating to level of sexual development are linked to activity levels. Administered biochemical agents are well recognized for altering motor activity. Central nervous system lesions in animals alter activity energy expenditure, and disease states in humans characterized by hyperactivity have a biological basis. Neurochemical factors in the central nervous system have been identified that modulate physical activity. Rhythmic variability characteristic of biological systems is evident in physical activity behavior. A considerable hereditary influence on habitual activity levels has been documented, and specific gene loci have been identified that affect regular physical activity habits. The ubiquitous nature of play in the animal kingdom, including human children, speaks to a biological basis for this apparently purposeless activity.

Part II presents a reasonable rationale for such intrinsic regulation—that a biological controller of activity exists on an evolutionary basis as a participant in the stabilization of energy balance. It is logical that such a controller would function not as an isolated feedback system (i.e., via an activity-stat) but rather within the global context of balancing all the contributors to the energy balance equation (i.e., subservient to an overencompassing energy-stat). This part proposes a plausible mechanistic construct for a feedback homeostatic system of control of physical activity based on previously established elements in other such systems.

Although this information bears credibility, it does—as forewarned in the preface—raise a good deal more questions than answers. Part III raises the unresolved issues surrounding considerations of compensatory responses to perturbation of energy balance, particularly those involving the etiology of human obesity. Many questions are identified that, in fact, remain unresolved. What is the role of hedonistic behaviors in affecting energy balance? How important is NEAT in this picture? What is the relative importance of intrinsic biologic versus environmental extrinsic factors in establishing level of physical activity behavior? How should strategies for promoting behavior be designed—both on an individual and population-wide basis—in respect to these influences? Can interventions for improving habits of physical activity be formulated involving environmental and biologic determinants of activity that operate in concert with each other?

Perhaps there is only one truly confident conclusion that can be drawn here: These issues bear a great deal of importance in defining the most appropriate and effective efforts for improving the physical activity habits of the population for salutary health outcomes. Consequently, future investigative efforts are warranted in a quest for filling in the many gaps in the understanding of the nature and implications of biological control of physical activity. To wit:

• Experimental research designs for examining activity determinants need to incorporate accurate measures of activity energy expenditure. For the most part, this means the employment of *objective* measures of physical activity, such as accelerometry and doubly labeled water. Most previous studies have relied on self-report of activity, an approach that often lacks accuracy and that is influenced by reporter bias. On the other hand, as Telama observed in respect to tracking studies, "although objective methods measure physical activity more accurately during the measurement itself, their ability to capture a sufficient sample of the individual's activity or day-to-day variation may be lower than that of self-report. Recording usually covers a few days or, at most, 1 week. The self-report method in turn may better capture on various activities, including, for instance, seasonal variation, but involves a larger measurement error than is the case in objective methods" (70, p. 191).

• Research investigations of energy balance need to include concomitant assessment of all contributing elements to energy intake and expenditure. Any measurement of compensation of one factor after perturbation of another needs to be performed over extended periods (62). There is evidence to suspect that such adaptations are not immediate, yet the time frame to be considered is not currently known. Moreover, differences among individuals in the rapidity and magnitude of such compensations may prove to bear importance in explaining interindividual variations in body weight changes in the face of energy imbalance.

• Frequently lost in the research literature on determinants of physical activity is the influence of intra- and interindividual variability (62). Outcomes are reported as group means, which can identify biological trends but say nothing about the level of predictability of such an outcome and its magnitude in a given individual. Limited information suggests, in fact, that such variability may be wide. As Claude Bernard wrote forcefully in 1865, "An average description of symptoms observed in individual cases [will create] a description that will never be matched in nature. So in physiology, we must never make average descriptions of experiments, because the true relations of phenomena disappear in the average" (5, p. 135). The effect of this "tyranny of the mean" is that little information can be expected to be derived regarding responses of individual people to perturbations of energy balance by considering average values and experimental outcomes. For the clinician in an ambulatory clinic advising lifestyle interventions to an obese teenager, this challenge of recognizing expected treatment outcomes has real meaning.

• The recent development of neuroimaging techniques to identify metabolically active regions of the central nervous system may provide key information regarding neurologic determinants of physical activity. For example, localization of centers affecting spontaneous activity versus hedonistic activity in both animals and humans would prove of interest, particularly in response to excessive caloric intake. Although many are excited about the potential of such technology to discern areas of the brain responsible for, say, the urge to participate in physical activity, skeptics also exist (26). The latter would argue that mental activities are generally performed by networks of intercommunicating areas of the brain, not a single geographical site. And the lighting up of areas on a brain scan during a particular action only "adds a false gloss of scientific certainty" when attempting to decipher brain functions (26, p. 87).

• More in-depth studies of contemporary hunter-gatherer societies that are currently living in isolation from the obesogenic high-calorie, low-activity existence of advanced cultures would provide insights regarding how the energy balance system might have functioned during prehistoric times. Such investigations could examine, for instance, the common assumption that evolutionary pressures existed for conditions of negative rather than positive caloric balance. In addition, an assessment of how daily energy expenditure might change over the life span of such societies would aid in sorting out the relative contributions of extrinsic and intrinsic factors in the decline of activity with age observed in contemporary populations.

• The potential for developing pharmaceutical agents with the capacity to repair or replace dysfunctional biochemical messengers in the energy balance system and regulate balance set points needs to be explored further. As Keesey and Hirvonen commented, "This is to suggest that future obesity research should have as an aim, first, the identification of factors responsible for setting the level at which such individuals regulate body weight and, second, the application of this knowledge to the design of procedures that would allow the system set-point to be readjusted" (33, p. 1880S).

• The multiplicity of scientific domains that have interest in the biological regulation of physical activity is obvious. The problem here is that neuro-chemists rarely talk with epidemiologists, and it is an uncommon molecular geneticist who meets regularly with the physicians in the outpatient obesity clinic. A greater efficiency in resolving the many questions surrounding the factors that control physical activity can be expected with increased efforts at interdisciplinary communication and collaboration.

One of the difficulties—and frustrations—in considering the nature and implications of a biological regulator of physical activity is explaining conflicting research outcomes: Half of experimental studies demonstrate a compensatory decrease in nonexercise physical activity after an activity intervention; another half do not. And findings seem contrary to expecta-tions: Dietary caloric intake does not, in most studies, increase in response to programs of physical activity. Physiologic findings are puzzling: Why should leptin operate differently in human beings than in other animals?

Although these conundrums are not truly errors, they might be considered in the same way that Craver and Darden suggested one should view expected outcomes in research that turn out to be untrue:

The engine of mechanism discovery is in many cases fueled not by experimental success, in which a prized mechanism schema is con-firmed by careful observation and experiment, but by failures in which the prized schema turns out to contain an error. So while there is a tendency to despair at moments when the world does not cooperate with our favored schemas, such failures are also a cause for celebration: failures often contain within them clues that guide the construction of more plausible schemas. Understanding just how they fail is often a first step in building better schemas. (19, p. 144)

References

Preface

1. Burton RA. *A Skeptic's Guide to the Mind.* New York: St. Marin's Griffin; 2013.
2. Hallinan JT. *Why We Make Mistakes.* New York: Broadway Books; 2009.
3. Lehrer J. *How We Decide.* Boston: Mariner Books; 2009.
4. Libet B. *Mind Time. The Temporal Factor in Consciousness.* Cambridge, MA: Harvard University Press; 2004.
5. Rowland TW. The biological basis of physical activity. *Med Sci Sports Exerc.* 1998;30:392-399.
6. Rowland TW. Promoting physical activity for children's health. *Sports Med.* 2007;36:929-936.
7. Rowland TW. *The Athlete's Clock.* Champaign, IL: Human Kinetics; 2011.

Introduction

1. Borer KT. Nonhomeostatic control of human appetite and physical activity in regulation of energy balance. *Exerc Sport Sci Rev.* 2010;38:114-121.
2. Byers JA. The biology of human play. *Child Develop.* 1998;69:599-600.
3. Craver CF, Darden L. *In Search of Mechanisms. Discoveries Across the Life Sciences.* Chicago: University of Chicago Press; 2013.
4. Eaton SB, Eaton SB. An evolutionary perspective on human physical activity: Implication for health. *Comp Biochem Physiol.* 2003;136:153-159.
5. Eaton SB, Konner M, Shostak M. Stone Agers in the fast lane: Chronic degenerative diseases in evolutionary perspective. *Am J Med.* 1988;84:739-749.
6. Engel AK. Dynamic predictions: Oscillations and synchrony in top-down processing. *Nature Rev.* 2001;2:704-716.
7. Gopnik A. Mindless. *The New Yorker.* September 9, 2013: 86-88.
8. Hoar HS. *General Comparative Physiology.* 2nd ed. Englewood, NJ: Prentice-Hall; 1975.
9. Kennedy GC, Mitra J. Hypothalamic control of energy balance and the reproductive cycle in the rat. *J Physiol.* 1963;166:396-407.
10. Lehrer J. *How We Decide.* Boston: Mariner Books; 2009.

11. Levine JA, Kotz CM. NEAT—non-exercise activity thermogenesis— egocentric & geocentric environmental vs. biological regulation. *Acta Physiol Scand.* 2005;184:309-318.
12. Luiten PGM, ter Horst GJ, Steffens AB. The hypothalamus, intrinsic connection and outflow pathways to the endocrine system in relation to the control of feeding and metabolism. *Progr Neurobiol.* 1987;28:1-53.
13. Malina RM, Little BB. Physical activity: The present in the context of the past. *Am J Hum Biol.* 2008;20:373-391.
14. Noble D. *The music of life. Biology beyond the genome.* Oxford: Oxford University Press; 2006.
15. Nolte J. *The Human Brain. An Introduction to Its Functional Anatomy.* 6th ed. Philadelphia: Mosby; 2009.
16. Rowland T. *The Athlete's Clock.* Champaign, IL: Human Kinetics; 2011.
17. Sallis JF, Prochaska JJ, Taylor WC. A review of correlates of physical activity of children and adolescents. *Med Sci Sports Exerc.* 2000;32:963-975.
18. Schaeffer PJ, Lindstedt SL. How animals move: Comparative lessons on animal locomotion. *Compr Physiol.* 2013;3:289-314.
19. Schartz MW, Woods SC, Porte DJ, Seely RJ, Baskin DG. Central nervous system control of food intake. *Nature.* 2000;404:661-671.
20. Vogel S. *Comparative Biomechanics.* Princeton, NJ: Princeton University Press; 2003.

Part I

1. Adan RAH, Hillebrand JJG, Danner UN, Cano SC, Kas MJH, Verhagen LAW. Neurobiology driving hyperactivity in activity-based anorexia. In: Adan RAH, Kaye WH, eds. *Behavioral Neurobiology of Eating Disorders.* Heidelberg: Springer Verlag; 2010: 229-250.
2. Aldis O. *Play Fighting.* New York: Academic Press; 1975.
3. Almli CR, Ball RH, Wheeler ME. Human fetal and neonatal movement patterns: Gender differences and fetal-to-neonatal continuity. *Dev Psychobiol.* 2001;38:252-273.
4. Annemiek MCP, Joosen M, Gielen M, Vlietnick R, Westerterp KR. Genetic analysis of physical activity in twins. *Am J Clin Nutr.* 2005;82:1253-1259.
5. Arkhipkin A. Age, growth and maturation of the European squid *Loligo vulgaris* (Myopsida, Loliginidae) on the west Saharan shelf. *J Marine Biol Assoc Unit King.* 1995;75:593-604.
6. Atkinson G, Edwards B, Reilly T, Waterhouse J. Exercise as a synchronizer of human circadian rhythms: An update and discussion of the methodological problems. *Eur J Appl Physiol.* 2007:99:331-341.

7. Barron AB, Søvik E, Cornish JL. The roles of dopamine and related compounds in reward-seeking behavior across animal phyla. *Front Behav Neurosci.* 2010;4:163.
8. Barry VC, Klawans HL. On the role of dopamine in the pathophysiology of anorexia nervosa. *J Neural Transm.* 1976;38:107-122.
9. Beard JL. Neuroendocrine alterations in iron deficiency. *Progr Food Nutr Sci.* 1990;14:45-82.
10. Berman N, Bailey R, Barstow TJ, Cooper DM. Spectral and bout detection analysis of physical activity patterns in health prepubertal boys and girls. *Am J Hum Biol.* 1998;10:289-297.
11. Bijnen FCH, Feskens EJM, Caspersen CJ, Mosterd WL, Kromhout D. Age, period, and cohort effects on physical activity among elderly men during 10 years of follow-up: The Zutphen Elderly Study. *J. Gerontol.* 1998;53A:M235-M241.
12. Black AE, Coward WA, Cole TJ, Prentice AM. Human energy expenditure in affluent societies. *Eur J Clin Nutr.* 1996;50:72-92.
13. Bolanowski MA, Russell RL, Jacobson LA. Quantitative measures of aging in the nematode *Caenorhabditis elegans. Mech Ageing Dev.* 1981;15:279-295.
14. Bouchard C, Malina RM, Pérusse L. *Genetics of Fitness and Physical Performance.* Champaign, IL: Human Kinetics; 1997.
15. Bouchard C, Tremblay A. Genetic effects in human energy expenditure. *Int J Obes.* 1990;14(Suppl 1):49-58.
16. Bowen RS, Turner MJ, Lightfoot JT. Sex hormone effects on physical activity levels. Why doesn't Jane run as much as Dick? *Sports Med.* 2011;41:73-86.
17. Bronikowski AM, Rhodes JS, Garland TJ, Prolla TA, Awad TA, Gammie SC. The evolution of gene expression in mouse hippocampus in response to selective breeding for increased locomotor activity. *Evolution Int J Org Evolution.* 2004;58:2079-2086.
18. Budinich CS, Tucker LB, Lowe D, Rosenberger JG, McCabe JT. Short and long-term motor and behavioral effects of diazoxide and dimethyl sulfoxide administration in the mouse after traumatic brain injury. *Pharm Biochem Behav.* 2013;108(Suppl C):66-73.
19. Burton D. The dropout dilemma in youth sports: Documenting the problem and identifying solutions. In: Malina R, ed. *Young Athletes. Biological, Psychological and Educational Perspectives.* Champaign, IL: Human Kinetics; 1988: 245-266.
20. Butler AA, Cone RD. Knockout studies defining different roles of melanocortin receptors in energy homeostasis. *Ann NY Acad Sci.* 2003;994:240-245.

21. Butte NF, Treuth MS, Voight RG, Llorente AM, Heird WC. Stimulant medications decrease energy expenditure and physical activity with attention deficit/hyperactivity disorder. *J Pediatr.* 1999;135:203-207.
22. Byers JA, Walker C. Refining the motor training hypothesis for the evolution of play. *Am Nat.* 1995;146:25-40.
23. Cairney J, Veldhuizen S, Kwan M, Hay J, Faught BE. Biological age and sex-related declines in physical activity during adolescence. *Med Sci Sports Exerc.* 2013;46:730-735.
24. Campbell DW, Eaton WO. Sex differences in the activity level of infants. *Inf Child Develop.* 1999;8:1-17.
25. Carey N. *The Epigenetics Revolution.* New York: Columbia University Press; 2012.
26. Casper RC. The "drive for activity" and "restlessness" in anorexia nervosa: Potential pathways. *J Affect Disord.* 2006;92:99-107.
27. Caspersen CJ, Pereira MA, Curran KM. Changes in physical activity patterns in the United States, by sex and cross-sectional age. *Med Sci Sports Exerc.* 2000;32:1601-1609.
28. Caspersen CJ, Powell KE, Christenson GM. Physical activity, exercise, and physical fitness: Definitions and distinctions for health-related research. *Public Health Rep.* 1985;100:126-131.
29. Connor JR, Wang X-S, Allen RP, Beard JL, Wiesinger JA, Felt BT, Earley CJ. Altered dopaminergic profile in the putamen and substantia nigra in restless leg syndrome. *Brain.* 2009;132:2403-2412.
30. Cooper DM, Bailey RC, Barstow TJ, Berman N. Spectral analysis of spontaneous patterns of physical activity in children [abstract]. *Med Sci Sports Exerc.* 1995;27(Suppl): S165.
31. Corder K, Ekelund U. Physical activity. In: Armstrong N, van Mechelen W, eds. *Paediatric Exercise Science and Medicine.* Oxford: Oxford University Press; 2008: 129-143.
32. Cumming SP. New directions in the study of maturation and physical activity. In: Katzmarzyk PT, Coelho e Silva MJ, eds. *Growth and Maturation in Human Biology and Sports.* Coimbra, Portugal: Imprensada Universidade de Coimbra; 2013: 129-138.
33. Cumming SP, Sherar LB, Esliger DW, Riddoch CJ, Malina RM. Concurrent and prospective associations among biological maturation and physical activity at 11 and 13 years of age. *Scand J Med Sci Sports.* 2014;24:e20-e28.
34. Cumming SP, Standage M, Gillison F, Malina RM. Sex differences in exercise behavior during adolescence: Is biological maturation a confounding factor? *J Adol Health.* 2011;34:465-473.

35. Dantas RAE, Passos KE, Porto LB, Zakir JCO, Reis MC, Naves LA. Physical activities in daily life and functional capacity compared to disease activity control in acromegalic patients: Impact in self-reported quality of life. *Arq Bras Endocrinol Metabl.* 2013;57(7): 550-557.

36. Dauvilliers Y, Winkelmann J. Restless leg syndrome: Uptake on pathogenesis. *Curr Opin Pulm Med.* 2013;19:594-600.

37. Davis C. Eating disorders and hyperactivity: A psychobiological perspective. *Can J Psychiatry.* 1997;42:168-175.

38. Davis C, Claridge G. The eating disorders as addiction: A psychobiological perspective. *Addict Behav.* 1998;23:463-475.

39. Del Bel EA. Role of nitric oxide on motor behavior. *Cell Mol Neurobiol.* 2005;25:371-392.

40. DeMoor MHM, Liu Y-J, Boomsma DI, Li J, Hamilton JJ, Hottenga J-J, Levy S, et al. Genome-wide association study of exercise behavior in Dutch and American adults. *Med Sci Sports Exerc.* 2009;41:1887-1895.

41. Dumuth D, Gigante D, Domingues M, Kohl HW. Physical activity change during adolescence: A systematic review and a pooled analysis. *Int J Epidemiol.* 2011;40:685-698.

42. Dunlap JC, Loros JJ, DeCoursey PJ, eds. *Biological Timekeeping.* Sunderland, MA: Sinauer; 2004.

43. Eaton WO, Enns LR. Sex differences in human motor activity level. *Psychol Bull.* 1986;100:19-28.

44. Eaton WO, Yu AP. Are sex differences in child motor activity a function of sex differences in maturational status? *Child Dev.* 1989;60:1005-1011.

45. Eisenmann JC, Wickel EE. The biological basis of physical activity in children: Revisited. *Pediatr Exerc Science.* 2009;21:257-272.

46. Ekbom K, Ulkberg J. Restless legs syndrome. *J Intern Med.* 2009;266:419-431.

47. Ellacott KL, Cone RD. The central melanocortin system and the integration of short- and long-term regulators of energy homeostasis. *Recent Prog Horm Res.* 2004;59:395-408.

48. Ellis MJ, Wade MG, Bohrer RE. Short biorhythms in children's play. Presented at the annual meeting of the Canadian Association for Health, Physical Education and Recreation, Waterloo, Ontario, 1971.

49. Eriksson M, Rasmussen F, Tynelius P. Genetic factors in physical activity and equal environment assumption—the Swedish young male twins study. *Behav Genet.* 2006;36:238-247.

50. Fagen R. *Animal Play Behavior.* New York: Oxford University Press; 1981.

51. Fifel K, Vezoli J, Dzahini K, Claustrat B, Leviel V, Kennedy H, Procyk E, et al. Alteration of daily and circadian rhythms following dopamine depletion in MPTP treated non-human primates. *PLoS One.* 2014;9:e86240.

52. Fink JS, Reis DJ. Genetic variation in midbrain dopamine cell number: Parallel with differences in responses to dopaminergic agonists and in naturalistic behaviors mediated by central dopaminergic systems. *Brain Res.* 1981;222:335-349.

53. Foley TE, Greenwood BN, Day HE, Koch LG, Britton SL, Fleshner M. Elevated central monoamine receptor mRNA in rats bred for high endurance capacity: Implications for central fatigue. *Behav Brain Res.* 2006;174(1):132-142.

54. Franks PW, Ravussin E, Hanson RL, Harper IT, Allison DB, Knowler WC, et al. Habitual activity in children: The role of genes and the environment. *Am J Clin Nutr.* 2005;82:901-908.

55. Freedson PS, Melanson EL. Measuring physical activity. In: Docherty D, ed. *Measurement in Pediatric Exercise Science.* Champaign, IL: Human Kinetics; 1996: 261-284.

56. Garland T, Kelly SA. Phenotype plasticity and experimental evolution. *J Exp Biol.* 2006;209:2344-2361.

57. Garland T, Schutz H, Chappell MA, Keeney BK, Meek TH, Copes LE, Acosta W, et al. The biological control of voluntary exercise, spontaneous activity and daily energy expenditure in relation to obesity: Human and rodent perspectives. *J Exp Biol.* 2011;214:206-229.

58. Goncharov NP, Katsia GV, Dzholua AA, Barkaia VS, Kulava ZV, Mikvabia ZL. The influence of dehydroepiandrosterone (DHEA) on the behavior in old non-human primates [Russian]. *Fiziol Cheloveka.* 2014;40:41-48.

59. Harz KJ, Muller HL, Waldeck E, Pudel V, Roth C. Obesity in patients with craniopharyngioma: Assessment of food intake and movement counts indicating physical activity. *J Clin Endocrinol Metab.* 2003;88:5227-5231.

60. Hastings JE, Barkley RA. A review of psychophysiological research with hyperkinetic children. *J Abnorm Child Psych.* 1978;6:413-447.

61. Head E, Callahan H, Cummings BJ, Cotman CW, Ruehl WW, Muggenberg BA, Milgram NW. Open field activity and human interaction as a function of age and breed in dogs. *Physiol Behav.* 1997;62:963-971.

62. Huppertz C, Meike B, Broen-Blokhuis MM, Dolan CV, de Moor MHM, Abellaoui A, van Beijsterveldt CEM, et al. The dopamine reward system and leisure time exercise behavior: A candidate allele study. *Biomed Res Int.* 2014;2014:591717.

63. Hwa JJ, Ghibaudi L, Gao J, Parker EM. Central melanocortin system modulates energy intake and expenditure of obese and lean Zucker rats. *Am J Physiol Reg Int Comp Physiol.* 2001;281:R444-R451.

64. Ingram DK. Age-related decline in physical activity: Generalization to nonhumans. *Med Sci Sports Exerc.* 2000;32:1623-1629.

65. Iwamoto GA, Wappel S, Fox GM, Buetow KA, Waldrop TG. Identification of diencephalic and brainstem cardiorespiratory areas activated during exercise. *Brain Research.* 1996;726:109-122.

66. Janicke B, Coper D, Janicke UA. Motor activity of different-aged Cercopithecidae: Silver-leafed monkey (*Presbytis cristatus* esch.), lion-tailed monkey (*Macaca silenus L.*), moor macaque (*Macaca maura Cuv.*) as observed in the zoological garden. *Gerontology.* 1986;32:133-140.

67. Jéquier E. Leptin signaling, adiposity, and energy balance. *Ann NY Acad Sci.* 2002;967-988.

68. Johnson MS. Effect of continuous light on periodic spontaneous activity in white-footed mice. *J Exp Zool.* 1939;82:315-328.

69. Kaprio J, Koskenvuo M, Sarna S. Cigarette smoking, use of alcohol, and leisure time physical activity among same-sexed adult male twins. In: Gedda L, Parisi P, Nance WE, eds. *Progress in Clinical and Biological Research. Twin Research 3: Epidemiological and Clinical Studies.* New York: Liss; 1981: 37-46.

70. Katzmarzyk PT. Physical activity and fitness with age, sex, and ethnic differences. In: Bouchard C, Blair SN, Haskell WL, eds. *Physical Activity and Health.* 2nd ed. Champaign, IL: Human Kinetics; 2012: 39-51.

71. Kelly SA, Nehrenberg DL, Pierce JL, Hua K, Steffy BM, Wiltshire T, de Villena F, et al. Genetic architecture of voluntary exercise in an advanced intercross line of mice. *Physiol Genomics.* 2010;42: 190-200.

72. Kelly SA, Pomp D. Genetic determinants of voluntary exercise. *Trends Gen.* 2013;29:348-357.

73. Kieling C, Goncalves RRF, Tannock R, Castellanos FX. Neurobiology of attention deficit hyperactivity disorder. *Child Adolesc Psychiatric Clin N Amer.* 2009;17:285-307.

74. Kimm SYS, Glynn NW, Kriska AM, Fitzgerald SL, Aaron DJ, Similo SL, McMahon RP, Barton BA. Longitudinal changes in physical activity in a biracial cohort during adolescence. *Med Sci Sports Exerc.* 2000;32:1445-1454.

75. Knab AM, Bowen RS, Hamilton AT, Gulledge AA, Lightfoot JT. Altered dopaminergic profiles: Implications for the regulation of voluntary physical activity. *Behav Brain Res.* 2009;204:147-152.

76. Knab AM, Lightfoot JT. Does the difference between physically active and couch potato lie in the dopamine system? *Int J Biol Sci.* 2010;6:133-150.

77. Kohl M, Foulon C, Guelfi JD. Hyperactivity and anorexia nervosa: Behavioral and biological perspective [French]. *Encephale.* 2004;30:492-499.

78. Kontis D, Theochari E. Dopamine in anorexia nervosa: A systematic review. *Behav Pharmacol.* 2012;23:496-515.

79. Kostrzewa E, Kas MJ. The use of mouse models to unravel genetic architecture of physical activity: A review. *Genes Brain Behav.* 2014;13:87-103.

80. Kotz CM, Teske JA, Billington CJ. Neuroregulation of nonexercise activity thermogenesis and obesity resistance. *Am J Physiol Integr Comp Physiol.* 2008;294:R699-R710.

81. Kotz CM, Wang C, Teske JA, Thorpe AJ, Novak CM, Kiwaki K, Levine JA. Orexin A mediation of time spent moving in rats: Neural mechanisms. *Neuroscience.* 2006;142(1):29-36.

82. Kron L, Katz JL, Weiner H. Hyperactivity in anorexia nervosa: A fundamental feature. *Compr Psychiatry.* 1978;19:433-440.

83. Lamont EW, Burton J, Blum ID, Abizaid A. Ghrelin receptor-knockout mice display alterations in circadian rhythms of activity and feeding under constant lighting conditions. *Eur J Neurosci.* 2014;39: 207-217.

84. LeBourg E, Lints FA. Hypergravity and aging in Drosophila melanogaster. 5. Patterns of movement. *Gerontology.* 1992;38:65-70, 19912.

85. Levine JA, Kotz CM. NEAT—non-exercise activity thermogenesis—egocentric and geocentric environmental factors vs. biological regulation. *Acta Physiol Scand.* 2005;184:309-318.

86. Lhotellier L, Cogen-Salmon C. Genetics and senescence. 1. Age-related changes in activity and exploration in three inbred strains of mice. *Physiol Behav.* 1989;45:491-493.

87. Lightfoot JT. Sex hormones' regulation of rodent physical activity: A review. *Int J Biol Sci.* 2008;4:126-132.

88. Lightfoot JT. Current understanding of the genetic basis for physical activity. *J Nutr.* 2011;141:526-530.

89. Lightfoot JT, Leamy L, Pomp D, Turner MJ, Fodor AA, Knab A, Bowen RS, et al. Strain screen and haplotype association mapping of wheel running in inbred mouse strains. *J Appl Physiol.* 2010;109:623-634.

90. Liste I, Guerra MJ, Caruncho HJ, Labandera-Barcia JL. Treadmill running induces striatal FOS expression via NMDA glutamate and dopamine receptors. *Exp Brain Res.* 1997;115:458-468.

91. Liston C, Malter Cohen M, Teslovich T, Levenson D, Casey BJ. Atypical prefrontal connectivity in attention-deficit/hyperactivity disorder: Pathway to disease or pathological end point? *Biol Psychiatry.* 2011;69:1168-1177.

92. Madras BK, Miller GM, Fischman AJ. The dopamine transporter and attention-deficit/hyperactivity disorder. *Biol Psychiatry.* 2005;57:1397-1409.

93. Maia JA, Thomis M, Beunen G. Genetic factors in physical activity levels: A twin study. *Am J Prev Med.* 2002;23:87-91.

94. Malina RM, Little BB. Physical activity: The present in the context of the past. *Am J Hum Biol.* 2008;20:373-391.

95. Malina R. Biocultural factors in developing physical activity levels. In: Smith AL, Biddle SJH, eds. *Youth Physical Activity and Sedentary Behavior.* Champaign, IL: Human Kinetics; 2008: 141-166.

96. Malina RM, Bouchard C. *Growth, Maturation, and Physical Activity.* Champaign, IL:uman Kinetics, 1991I Human Kinetics; 1991: 3-10.

97. Marcheva B, Ramsey KM, Peek CB, Affinati A, Maury E, Bass J. Circadian clocks and metabolism. *Handb Exp Pharmacol.* 2013;217:127-155.

98. Marcus B, Gillette PC, Garson A. Intrinsic heart rate in children and young adults: An index of sinus node function isolated from autonomic control. *Am Heart J.* 1990;112:911-916.

99. Mathes WF, Aylor DL, Miller DR, Churchill GA, Chester EJ, de Villena FP, Threadgill DW, et al. Architecture of energy balance traits in emerging lines of the Collaborative Cross. *Am J Physiol Endocrinol Metab.* 2011;300:E1124-E1134.

100. Matthews CE, Freedson PS, Hebert JR, Stanek EJ, Merriam PA, Rosal MC, Ebbeling CB, et al. Season variation in household, occupational, and leisure time physical activity: Longitudinal analyses from the season variation of blood cholesterol study. *Am J Epidemiol.* 2001;153:172-183.

101. McMurray RG, Harrell JS, Bangdiwala SI, Hu J. Tracking of physical activity and aerobic power from childhood through adolescence. *Med Sci Sports Exerc.* 2003;35:1914-1922.

102. Meijer JH, Robbers Y. Wheel running in the wild. *Proc R Soc B.* 2014;281:1-5.

103. 103. Mooij-van Malsen JG, van Lith HA, Oppelaar OB, Kas MJH. Evidence for epigenetic interactions for loci on mouse chromosome 1 regulating open field activity. *Behav Genet.* 2009;39:176-182.

104. Naylor H, Mountford V, Brown G. Beliefs about excessive exercise in eating disorders: The role of obsessions and compulsions. *Eur Eat Disord Rev.* 2011;19:226-236.

105. Nilsson A, Brage S, Riddoch C, Anderssen SA, Sardinha LB, Wedderkopp N, Andersen LB, Ekelund U. Comparison of equations for predicting energy expenditure from accelerometer counts. *Scand J Med Sci Sports*. 2008;18:643-650.

106. Nisembaum LG, de Pedro N, Delgado MJ, Sanchez-Bretano A, Isorna E. Orexin as an input of circadian system in goldfish: Effects on clock gene expression and locomotor activity rhythms. *Peptides*. 2014;52:29-37.

107. Novak CM, Burghardt PR, Levine JA. The use of a running wheel to measure activity in rodents: Relationship to energy balance, general activity, and reward. *Neurosci Biobehav Rev*. 2012;36:1001-1014.

108. Oladehin A, Waters RS. Location and distribution of FOS protein expression in rat hippocampus following acute moderate aerobic exercise. *Exper Brain Res*. 2001;137:26-35.

109. Orsey AD, Wakefield DB, Cloutier MM. Physical activity (PA) and sleep among children and adolescents with cancer. *Pediatr Blood Cancer*. 2013;60:1908-1913.

110. Panksepp J, Siviy S, Normansell L. The psychobiology of play: Theoretical and methodological perspectives. *Neurosci Biobehav Rev*. 1984;8:465-492.

111. Pellegrini AD, Smith PK. Physical activity play: The nature and function of a neglected aspect of play. *Child Develop*. 1998;69: 577-598.

112. Perusse L, Tremblay A, Leblanc C, Bouchard C. Genetic and environmental influences on level of habitual physical activity and exercise participation. *Am J Epidemiol*. 1989;129:1012-1022.

113. Pfeiffer KA, Schmitz KH, McMurray RG, Treuth MS, Murray MS, Pate R. Physical activities in adolescent girls: Variability in energy expenditure. *Am J Prev Med*. 2006;31:328-331.

114. Prince J. Catecholamine dysfunction in attention-deficit/hyperactivity disorder: An update. *J Clin Psychopharmacol*. 2008;28(Suppl 2):S39-S45.

115. Prober DA. Hypocretin/orexin over-expression induces an insomnia-like phenotype in zebrafish. *J Neurosci*. 2006;26:13400-13410.

116. Ramsey KM, Bass J. Circadian clocks in fuel harvesting and energy homeostasis. *Cold Spring Harb Symp Quant Biol*. 2011;76:63-72.

117. Rhodes JS, Garland T, Gammie SC. Patterns of brain activity associated with variation in voluntary wheel-running behavior. *Behav Neurosci*. 2003;117:1243-1256.

118. Riley JL, Robinson ME, Wise EA. A meta-analytic review of pain perception across the menstrual cycle. *Pain*. 1999;81:225-235.

119. Rising R, Harper IT, Fontvielle AM, Ferraro RT, Spraul M, Ravussin E. Determinants of total energy expenditure: Variability in physical activity. *Am J Clin Nutr.* 1994;59:800-804.

120. Robles de Medina PG, Visser GH, Huizink AC, Buitelaar JK, Mulder EJ. Fetal behavior does not differ between boys and girls. *Early Hum Devel.* 2003;7:17-26.

121. Roth GS, Joseph JA. Cellular and molecular mechanisms of impaired dopamine function with aging. *Ann N Y Acad Sci.* 1994;719: 129-135.

122. Rowland T. Adolescence: A "risk factor" for physical inactivity. *Pres Council Phys Fitn Sports Res Dig.* 1999;3:1-5.

123. Rowland T. Inferior exercise economy in children: Perpetuating a myth? *Ped Exerc Sci.* 2012;24:501-506.

124. Rowland T, Staab J, Unnithan VB, Rambusch JM, Siconolfi SF. Mechanical efficiency during cycling in prepubertal and adult males. *Int J Sports Med.* 1990;11:452-455.

125. Roy EJ, Wade GN. Role of estrogens in androgen-induced spontaneous activity in male rats. *J Comp Physiol Psychol.* 1975;89:573-579.

126. Sallis JF, Buono MJ, Roby JJ, Micale FG, Nelson JA. Seven-day recall and other physical activity self-reports in children and adolescents. *Med Sci Sports Exerc.* 1993;25:99-108.

127. Sanchez-Gomar F, Garcia-Gimenez JL, Perez-Quilis C, Gomez-Cabrera MC, Pallardo FV, Lippi G. Physical exercise as an epigenetic modulator: Eustress, the "positive stress" as an effector of gene expression. *J Strength Cond Res.* 2012;26:3469-3472.

128. Saris WHM, Elvers JWH, van't Hof MA, Binkhorst RA. Changes in physical activity of children aged 6 to 12 years. In: Rutenfranz J, Mocellin R, Klimt F, eds. *Children and Exercise XII.* Champaign, IL: Human Kinetics; 1986: 121-130.

129. Saris WHM, van Erp-Baart MA, Brouns F, Westerterp K, ten Hoor F. Study on food intake and energy expenditure during extreme sustained exercise: The Tour de France. *Int J Med.* 1989;10:S26-S31.

130. Satterfield JH, Cantwell DP, Satterfield BT. Pathophysiology of the hyperactive child syndrome. *Arch Gen Psychiatry.* 1974;31: 839-844.

131. Schendzielorz J, Stengl M. Candidates for the light entrainment pathway to the circadian clock of the Madeira cockroach Rhyparobia maderae. *Cell Tissue Res.* 2014;355:447-462.

132. Sherar LB, Cumming SP, Eisenmann JC, Baxter-Jones ADG, Malina RM. Adolescent biological maturity and physical activity: Biology meets behavior. *Pediatr Exerc Science.* 2010;22:332-349.

133. Sherar LB, Esliger DW, Baxter-Jones ADG, Tremblay MS. Age and gender differences in youth physical activity: Does physical maturity matter? *Med Sci Sports Exerc.* 2007;39:830-835.

134. Silbergeld EK, Goldberg AM. Hyperactivity: A lead-induced behavior disorder. *Environ Health Perspect.* 1974;34:227-232.

135. Starling RD. Energy expenditure and aging: Effects of physical activity. *Int J Sport Nutr Exerc Metab.* 2001;11:S208-S217.

136. Starling RD, Toth MJ, Matthews DE, Poehlman ET. Energy requirements and physical activity of older free-living African Americans: A doubly labeled water study. *J Clin Endocrinol Metabol.* 1998;83:1529-1534.

137. Storey KB, Storey JM. Metabolic rate depression and biochemical adaptation in anaerobiosis, hibernation and estivation. *Quart Rev Biol.* 1990;65:145-173.

138. Stubbe JH, Boomsma DI, Vink JM. Genetic influences on exercise participation: A comparative study in adult twin samples from seven countries. *PLoS ONE.* 2006;1:e22.

139. Suzuki T, Ishikawa A, Nishimura M, Yoshimura T, Namikawa T, Ebihara S. Mapping quantitative trait loci for circadian behavioral rhythms in SMXA recombinant inbred strains. *Behav Genetics.* 2000;30:447-453.

140. Taylor GT. Fighting in juvenile rats and the ontogeny of agonistic behavior. *J Comp Physiol Psychol.* 1980;94:953-961.

141. Telama R, Yang X. Decline of physical activity from youth to young adulthood in Finland. *Med Sci Sports Exerc.* 2000;32:1617-1622.

142. Teske JA, Billington CJ, Kotz CM. Neuropeptidergic mediators of spontaneous physical activity and non-exercise activity thermogenesis. *Neuroendocrinology.* 2008;87:71-90.

143. Thompson AM, Baxter-Jones ADG, Mirwald RL, Bailey DA. Comparison of physical activity in male and female children: Does maturation matter? *Med Sci Sports Exerc.* 2003;35:1684-1690.

144. Thorburn AW, Proietto J. Biological determinants of spontaneous physical activity. *Obes Rev.* 2000;1:87-94.

145. Tou JCL, Wade CE. Determinants affecting physical activity levels in animal models. *Exp Biol Med.* 2002;227:587-600.

146. Turin B. Energy requirements of children and adolescents. *Pub Health Nutr.* 2005;8:968-993.

147. Van Mechelen W, Twisk JWR, Post GB, Snel J, Kemper HCG. Physical activity of young people: The Amsterdam Longitudinal Growth and Health Study. *Med Sci Sports Exerc.* 2000;32:1610-1616.

148. Verschuur R, Kemper HCG. Habitual physical activity in Dutch teenagers measured by heart rate. In: Binkhorst RA, Kemper HCG,

Saris WHM, eds. *Children and Exercise XI.* Champaign, IL: Human Kinetics; 1985: 194-202.

149. Viggiano D. The hyperactive syndrome: Metanalysis of genetic alterations, pharmacological treatments and brain lesions which increase locomotor activity. *Behav Brain Res.* 2008;194:1-14.

150. Viggiano D, Ruocco LA, Arcieri S, Sadile AG. Involvement of norepinephrine in the control of activity and attentive processes in animal models of attention deficit hyperactivity disorder. *Neural Plast.* 2004;11:133-149.

151. de Vilhena e Santos DM, Katzmarzyk PT, Seabra AF, Maia JA. Genetics of physical activity and physical inactivity in humans. *Behav Genet.* 2012;42:559-578.

152. Wade MG, Ellis MJ, Bohrer RE. Biorhythms in the activity of children during free play. *J Exp Anal Behav.* 1973;20:155-162.

153. Waters RP, Renner KJ, Pringle RB, Summers CH, Britton SL, Koch LG, Swallow JG. Selection for aerobic capacity affects corticosterone, monoamines, and wheel-running activity. *Physiol Behav.* 2008:93:1044-1054.

154. West BJ. *Where Medicine Went Wrong. Rediscovering the Path to Complexity.* Singapore: World Scientific; 2006.

155. Westerterp KR, Plasqui G. Physical activity and human energy expenditure. *Curr Opin Clin Nutr Metab Care.* 2004;7:607-613.

156. Wolff G, Esser KA. Scheduled exercise phase shifts the circadian clock in skeletal muscle. *Med Sci Sports Exerc.* 2012;44:1663-1670.

157. Xiao L, Huang L, Schrack JA, Ferrucci L, Zipunnikov V, Crainiceanu CM. Quantifying the lifetime circadian rhythm of physical activity: a covariate-dependent functional approach. *Biostatistics.* 2015;16(2):352-367.

158. Zakeri I, Adolph AL, Puyau MR, Vohra FA, Butte NF. Application of cross-sectional time series modeling for the prediction of energy expenditure from heart rate and accelerometry. *J Appl Physiol.* 2008;104:1665-1673.

159. Zametkin AJ, Liotta W. The neurobiology of attention-deficit/hyperactivity disorder. *J Clin Psychiatry.* 1998;59(Suppl 7):17-23.

160. Zhang FF, Carderelli R, Carroll J, Zhang S, Fulda KG, Gonzalez K, Vishwanatha JK, et al. Physical activity and global genomic DNA methylation in a cancer-free population. *Epigenetics.* 2011;6:293-299.

161. Zou S, Liedo P, Altamirano-Robles L, Cruz-Enriquez J, Morice A, Ingram DK, Kraub J, Papadopoulos N, Carey JR. Recording lifetime behavior and movement in an invertebrate model. *PLoS ONE.* 2011;6:e18151.

Part II

1. Ahima RS. Revisiting leptin's role in obesity and weight loss. *J Clin Invest.* 2008;118:2380-2383.
2. Alpert SS. Growth, thermogenesis, and hyperphagia. *Am J Clin Nutr.* 1990;52:784-792.
3. Apfelbaum M, Bostsarron J, Lacatis D. Effect of caloric restriction and excessive caloric intake on energy expenditure. *Am J Clin Nutr.* 1971;24:1405-1409.
4. Bahr R, Ingnes I, Vaage O, Sejersted OM, Newshlme E. Effect of duration of exercise on O_2 consumption. *J Appl Physiol.* 1987;62:485-490.
5. Ballor DL. Exercise training elevates RMR during moderate but not severe dietary restriction in obese male rats. *J Appl Physiol.* 1991;70:2302-2310.
6. Ballor DL, Poehlman ET. A meta-analysis of the effects of exercise and/or dietary restriction on resting metabolic rate. *Eur J Appl Physiol.* 1995;71:535-42, 1995.
7. Ballor DL, Tommerup LJ, Thomas DP, Thomas DP, Smith DB, Keesey RE. Exercise training attenuates diet-induced reduction in metabolic rate. *J Appl Physiol.* 1990;68:2612-2617.
8. Batterham RL, Cohen MA, Ellis SM, LeRoux CW, Withers DJ, Frost GS, Ghatei MA, et al. Inhibition of food intake in obese subjects by peptide YY_{3-36}. *N Engl J Med.* 2003;349:941-948.
9. Benedict FG, Miles WR, Roth P, Smith HM. *Human vitality and efficiency under prolonged restricted diet.* Washington, DC: Carnegie Institute Washington, Publication No. 280; 1919.
10. Bernard C. *An Introduction to the Study of Experimental Medicine.* New York: Dover; 1957.
11. Bielinski R, Schutz Y, Jequier E. Energy metabolism during the postexercise recovery in man. *Am J Clin Nutr.* 1985;42:69-82.
12. Binzen CA, Swan PD, Manore MM. Postexercise oxygen consumption and substrate use after resistance exercise in women. *Med Sci Sports Exerc.* 2001;33:932-938.
13. Birkhead NC. Cardiodynamic and metabolic effects of prolonged bed rest. Dayton: AMRL-TDR-63-37, Wright-Patterson Air Force Base; 1963.
14. Blundell JE, King NA. Physical activity and regulation of food intake: Current evidence. *Med Sci Sports Exerc.* 1999;31(Suppl):S573-S583.
15. Blundell JE, Stubbs RJ, Hughes DA, Whybrow S, King NA. Cross talk between physical activity and appetite control: Does physical activity stimulate appetite? *Proc Nutr Soc.* 2003;62:651-661.

16. Borer K, Kaplan L. Exercise-induced growth in golden hamsters: Effects of age, weight, and activity levels. *Physiol Behav.* 1977;18:23-34.

17. Boström P, Wu J, Jedrychowski MP. A PGC-1\ga\-dependent myokine that drives brown fat-like development of white fat and thermogenesis. *Nature.* 2012;481:463-468.

18. Bouchard C, Tremblay A, Nadeau A. Genetic effect in resting and exercise metabolic rates. *Metabolism.* 1989;38:364-370.

19. Boushel R. Muscular metaboreflex control of the circulation during exercise. *Acta Physiol.* 2010:199:367-383.

20. Briefel RR, McDowell MA, Alaimo K. Total energy intake of the US population: The third National Health and Nutrition Examination Survey, 1988-1991. *Am J Clin Nutr.* 1995;62 (Suppl):1072S-1080S.

21. Butte NF, Moon JK, Wong WW, Hopkinson JM, O'Brian Smith E. Energy requirements from infancy to adulthood. *Am J Clin Nutr.* 1995;62(Suppl):1047S-1052S.

22. Byrne HK, Wilmore JH. The relationship of mode and intensity of training on resting metabolic rate in women. *Int J Sport Nutr Exerc Metab.* 2001;11:1-4.

23. Cannon WB. *The Wisdom of the Body.* New York: W.W. Norton; 1932.

24. Ceccarini G, Maffei M, Vitti P, Santini F. Fuel homeostasis and locomotor behavior: Role of leptin and melanocortin pathways. *J Endocrinol Invest.* 2015;38(2):125-131.

25. Craver CF, Darden L. *In Search of Mechanisms. Discoveries Across the Life Sciences.* Chicago: University of Chicago Press; 2013.

26. Crease RP, Goldhaber AS. *The Quantum Moment.* New York: W.W. Norton; 2014: 9-26.

27. Cuthbertson DP. The influence of prolonged muscular rest on metabolism. *Biochemistry.* 1929;23:1328-1345.

28. Danforth E. The role of thyroid hormones and insulin in the regulation of energy metabolism. *Am J Clin Nutr.* 1983;38:1006-1017.

29. Deitrick JE, Whedon GH, Shorr E. Effects of immobilization upon various metabolic and physiologic functions in normal man. *Am J Med.* 1948;4:3-36.

30. DeVries HA, Gray DE. Aftereffects of exercise upon resting metabolic rate. *Res Q.* 1963;34:314-321.

31. Dolezal BA, Potteiger JA, Jacobsen DJ, Benedict SH. Muscle damage and resting metabolic rate after acute resistance exercise with an eccentric overload. *Med Sci Sports Exerc.* 2000;32:1202-1207.

32. Donnelly JE, Herrmann SD, Lambourne K, Szabo AN, Honas JJ, Washburn RA. Does increased exercise or physical activity alter ad-libitum daily energy intake or macronutrient composition in healthy

adults? A systematic review. *PLoS ONE*. 2014;9:e83498. doi:10.371/journal.pone.0083498.

33. Edholm OG, Adam JM, Healy MJR, Wolff HS, Goldsmith R, Best TW. Food intake and energy expenditure of army recruits. *Br J Nutr*. 1970;24:1091-1107.

34. Edwards HT, Thorndike A, Dill DB. The energy requirement in strenuous muscular exercise. *N Engl J Med*. 1935;213:532-535.

35. Eisenmann JC, Wickel EE. The biologic basis of physical activity in children: Revisited. *Pediatr Exerc Science*. 2009;21:257-272.

36. Freymond D, Larson K, Bogardus C, Ravussin E. Energy expenditure during normo- and overfeeding in prepubertal children of lean and obese Pima Indians. *Am J Physiol*. 1989;257:E647-E653.

37. Garland T, Schutz H, Chappell MA, Keeney BK, Meek TH, Copes LE, Acosta W, et al. The biologic control of voluntary exercise, spontaneous physical activity and daily energy expenditure in relation to obesity: Human and rodent perspectives. *J Exper Biol*. 2011;214:206-229.

38. Gleeson M, Brown JF, Waring JJ, Stock MJ. The effects of physical activity on metabolic rate and dietary-induced thermogenesis. *Brit J Nutr*. 1982;47:173-181.

39. Gomersall SR, Rowlands AV, English C, Maher C, Olds TS. The ActivityStat hypothesis: The concept, the evidence, and the methodologies. *Sports Med*. 2013;43:135-149.

40. Goodner C, Ogilve J. Homeostasis of body weight in a diabetes clinic population. *Diabetes*. 1974;23:318-326.

41. Hall KD, Heymsfield SB, Kemnitz JW, Klein S, Schoeller DA, Speakman JR. Energy balance and its components: Implications for body weight regulation. *Am J Clin Nutr*. 2012;95:989-995.

42. Haralambie G. Activities enzymatiques dans le muscle squelettique des enfants de divers age [Enzymatic activities in the skeletal muscle of children of various ages]. In: *Les sports et l'enfant*. Montpelier, France: Euromed; 1980: 248-253.

43. Hill JO, Davis JR, Tagliaferro AR. Effects of diet and exercise training on thermogenesis in adult female rats. *Physiol Behav*. 1983;31: 133-135.

44. Hill JO, Davis JR, Tagliaferro AR, Stewart J. Dietary obesity and exercise in young rats. *Physiol Behav*. 1984;33:321-328.

45. Hill JO, Heymsfield SB, McMannus C, DiGirolamo M. Meal size and thermic response to food in male subjects as a function of maximum aerobic capacity. *Metabolism*. 1984;3:743-749.

46. Hill JO, Melby C, Johnson SL, Peters JC. Physical activity and energy requirements. *Am J Clin Nutr*. 1995;62(Suppl): 1059S-1066S.

47. Hirata K. Blood flow to brown adipose tissue and norepinephrine induced calorigenesis in physically trained rats. *Jpn J Physiol.* 1982;32:279-291.

48. Holliday MA, Potter D, Jarrah A, Bearg S. The relation of metabolic rate to body weight and organ size. *Pediatr Res.* 1967;1:185-195.

49. Houle-Leroy P, Guderley H, Swallow JG, Garland T. Artificial selection for high activity favors mighty mini-muscles in house mice. *Am J Physiol.* 2003;284:R433-R443.

50. Jéquier E. Leptin signaling, adiposity, and energy balance. *Ann NY Acad Sci.* 2002;967:379-388.

51. Keesey RE, Hirvonen MD. Body weight set points: Determination and adjustment. *J Nutr.* 1997;127:1875S-1883S.

52. Kersting M, Sichert-Hellert W, Lausen B, Alexy U, Manz F, Schoch G. Energy intake of 1 to 18 year old German children and adolescents. *Z Ernhrungswiss.* 1998;37:47-55.

53. Keys A, Brozek J, Henschel A, Michelsen O, Taylor HL. *The Biology of Human Starvation.* Minneapolis: University of Minnesota Press; 1950.

54. Khosa T, Billewicz WZ. Measurement of changes in body weight. *Br J Nutr.* 1964;18:227-239.

55. King NA, Caudwell P, Hopkins M, Byrne NM, Colley R, Hills AP, Stubbs JR, Blundell JE. Metabolic and behavioral compensatory responses to exercise interventions: Barriers to weight loss. *Obesity.* 2007;15:1373-1383.

56. Knoebel LK. Energy metabolism. In: Selkurt EE, ed. *Physiology.* Boston: Little Brown; 1963: 564-579.

57. Korner J, Leibel RL. To eat or not to eat—How the gut talks to the brain. *N Engl J Med.* 2003;349:926-928.

58. Landsberg L, Young JB. The role of the sympathetic nervous system and catecholamines in the regulation of energy metabolism. *Am J Clin Nutr.* 1983;38:1018-1024.

59. Lawson S, Webster JD, Pacy PJ, Garrow JS. Effect of a 10-week aerobic exercise programme on metabolic rate, body composition, and fitness in lean sedentary females. *Br J Clin Prac.* 1987;41:684-688.

60. LeBlanc J, Diamond P, Cote J, Labrie A. Hormonal factors in reduced postprandial heat production of exercise-training subjects. *J Appl Physiol.* 1984;56:772-776.

61. Leibel RL, Rosenbaum M, Hirsch J. Changes in energy expenditure resulting from altered body weight. *N Engl J Med.* 1995;332:621-628.

62. Lenart NR, Berthoud H-R. Central and peripheral regulation of food intake and physical activity: Pathways and genes. *Obesity.* 2008;16(Suppl 3):S11-S22.

63. Lightfoot JT. Why control activity? Evolutionary selection pressures affecting the development of physical activity genetic and biological regulation. *Biomed Res Int.* 2013;2013:82168.

64. Lin J, Handschin C, Spiegelman BM. Metabolic control through the PGC-1 family of transcription coactivators. *Cell Metab.* 2005;1:361-370.

65. Lortie G, Simoneau JA, Hamel P, Boulay MR, Landry F, Bouchard C. Responses of maximal aerobic power and capacity to aerobic training. *Int J Sports Med.* 1984;5:232-236.

66. Luiten PGM, ter horst GJ, Steffens AB. The hypothalamus, intrinsic connection and outflow pathways to the endocrine system in relation to the control of feeding and metabolism. *Progr Neurobiol.* 1987;28: 1-54.

67. Luke A, Schoeller DA. Basal metabolic rate, fat-free mass, and body cell mass during energy restriction. *Metab Clin Exper.* 1992;41:450-456.

68. Maehlum S, Grandmontagne M, Newsholme E, Sejersted M. Magnitude and duration of excess postexercise oxygen consumption in healthy young subjects. *Metabolism.* 1986;35:425-429.

69. Malina RM, Little BB. Physical activity: The present in the context of the past. *Am J Hum Biol.* 2008;20:373-391.

70. McArdle WD, Katch FI, Katch VL. *Exercise Physiology. Energy, Nutrition, and Human Performance.* Philadelphia: Lea & Febiger; 1981: 105-108.

71. McDonald RB, Wickler S, Horwitz B, Stern JS. Meal-induced thermogenesis following exercise training in the rat. *Med Sci Sports Exerc.* 1988;20:44-49.

72. McMurray RG, Soares J, Caspersen CJ, McCurdy T. Examining variations of resting metabolic rate of adults: A public health perspective. *Med Sci Sports Exerc.* 2014;46:1352-1358.

73. Melby C, Scholl C, Edwards G, Bullough R. Effect of acute resistance exercise on postexercise energy expenditure and resting metabolic rate. *J Appl Physiol.* 1993;75:1847-1853.

74. Melby CL, Tincknell T, Schmidt WD. Energy expenditure following a bout of unsteady state resistance exercise. *J Sports Med Phys Fitness.* 1992;32:128-135.

75. Molé PA. Impact of energy intake and exercise on resting metabolic rate. *Sports Med.* 1990;10:72-87.

76. Moore MS, Dodd CJ, Welsman JR, Armstrong N. Short-term appetite and energy intake following imposed exercise in 9- to 10-year-old girls. *Appetite.* 2004;43:127-134.

77. Moraska A, Deak T, Spencer RL, Roth D, Fleshner M. Treadmill running produces both positive and negative physiological adaptation in Sprague-Dawley rats. *Am J Physiol.* 2000;79:R1321-R1329.
78. Morgulis S. *Fasting and Undernutrition.* New York: Dutton; 1923: 1923.
79. Morton GJ. Hypothalamic leptin regulation of energy homeostasis and glucose metabolism. *J Physiol.* 2007;583:437-443.
80. Murphy MN, Mizuno M, Mitchell JH, Smith SA. Cardiovascular regulation by skeletal muscle reflexes in health and disease. *Am J Physiol Heart Circ Physiol.* 2011;301:H1191-H1204.
81. Nadel ER. Temperature regulation and hyperthermia during exercise. *Clin Chest Med.* 1984;5:13-20.
82. Pedersen BK. A muscular twist on the fate of fat. *N Engl J Med.* 2012;366:1544-1545.
83. Pinto ML, Shetty PS. Exercise induced changes in the energy expenditure of female Wistar rats. *Ind J Exper Biol.* 1995;33:105-108.
84. Poehlman ET. A review: Exercise and its influence on resting energy metabolism in man. *Med Sci Sports Exerc.* 1989;21:515-525.
85. Poehlman ET, LaChance P, Temblay A. The effect of prior exercise and caffeine ingestion on metabolic rate and hormones in young adult males. *Can J Physiol Pharmacol.* 1989;67:10-16.
86. Poehlman ET, Melby CL, Badylak SF. Resting metabolic rate and postprandial thermogenesis in highly trained and untrained males. *Am J Clin Nutr.* 1988;47:793-798.
87. Poehlman ET, Melby CL, Badylak SF, Calles J. Aerobic fitness and resting metabolic expenditure in young adult males. *Metabolism.* 1989;38:85-90.
88. Ravussin E, Lillioja S, Anderson TE, Christin L, Bogardus C. Determinants of 24-hour energy expenditure in man. *J Clin Invest.* 1986;78:1568-1578.
89. Redman LM, Ravussin E. Caloric restriction in humans: Impact on physiological, psychological, and behavioral outcomes. *Antioxid Redox Signal.* 2011;14:275-287.
90. Ridgers ND, Timperio A, Cerin E, Salmon J. Compensation of physical activity and sedentary time in primary school children. *Med Sci Sports Exerc.* 2014;46:1564-1569.
91. Rowland TW. *Developmental Exercise Physiology.* Champaign, IL: Human Kinetics; 1996.
92. Rowland TW. The childhood obesity epidemic: Putting the "dynamics" into thermodynamics. *Pediatr Exerc Science.* 2004;16:87-93.
93. Rubner M. Ueber den Einfluss der Korpergrosse auf Stoffund Kraftwechsel. *Z Biol.* 1883;19:535-562.

94. Rui L. Brain regulation of energy balance and body weights. *Rev Endocr Metab Disord.* 2013;14(4):387-407.

95. Saltin B, Hermansen L. Esophageal, rectal, and muscle temperature during exercise. *J Appl Physiol.* 1966;21:1757-1762.

96. Saris WHM, van Erp-Baart MA, Westerterp KR, ten Hoor F. Study on food intake and energy expenditure during extreme sustained exercise: The Tour de France. *Int J Sports Med.* 1989;10(Suppl 1): S26-S31.

97. Scharhag-Rosenberger F, Meyer T, Wegmann M, Ruppenthal S, Kaestner L, Morsch A, Hecksteden A. Irisin does not mediate resistance training-induced alterations in resting metabolic rate. *Med Sci Sports Exerc.* 2014;46:1736-1743.

98. Scharrer E, Langhans W. Metabolic and hormonal factors controlling food intake. *Internat J Vit Nutr Res.* 1988;58:249-261.

99. Schmidt-Nielsen K, *Scaling. Why Is Animal Size so Important?* Cambridge: Cambridge University Press; 1984: 56-74.

100. Schulz LO, Alger S, Harper I, Wilmore JH, Ravussin E. Energy expenditure of elite female runners measured by respiratory chamber and double labeled water. *J Appl Physiol.* 1992;72:23-28.

101. Schulz LO, Nyomba BL, Alger S, Anderson TW, Ravussin E. Effect of endurance training on sedentary energy expenditure measured in a respiratory chamber. *Am J Physiol.* 1991;260:E257-E261.

102. Schutz Y, Acheson KJ, Jequier E. Twenty-four hour energy expenditure and thermogenesis; response to progressive carbohydrate overfeeding in man. *Int J Obes.* 1985;9(Suppl 2):111-114.

103. Shibita H, Bukowiecki LJ. Regulatory alterations of daily energy expenditure induced by fasting or overfeeding unrestrained rats. *J Appl Physiol.* 1987;63:465-470.

104. Sjödin AM, Forslund AH, Westerterp KR, Andersson AB, Forslund JM, Hambraeus LM. The influence of physical activity on BMR. *Med Sci Sports Exerc.* 1996;28:85-91.

105. Speakman JR, Mitchell SE. Caloric restriction. *Mol Aspects Med.* 2011;32:159-221.

106. Speakman JR, Selman C. Physical activity and resting metabolic rate. *Proc Nutr Soc.* 2003;62:621-634.

107. Speakman JR, Westerterp KR. Associations between energy demands, physical activity, and body composition in adult humans between 18 and 96 y of age. *Am J Clin Nutr.* 2010;92:826-834.

108. Storey KB, Story JM. Metabolic rate depression and biochemical adaptation in anaerobiosis, hibernation and estivation. *Quart Rev Biol.* 1990;65:145-173

109. Stubbs RJ, Sepp A, Hughes DA, Johnstone AM, Horgan GW, King N, Blundell J. The effect of graded levels of exercise on energy intake and balance in free-living men, consuming their normal diet. *Eur J Clin Nutr.* 2002;56:129-140.

110. Tam CS, Ravussin E. Energy balance: An overview with emphasis on children. *Pediatr Blood Cancer.* 2012;58:154-158.

111. Tataranni PA, Gautier JF, Chen K, Uecker A, Bandy D, Salbe AD, Prately RE, et al. Neuroanatomical correlates of hunger and satiation in humans using positron emission tomography. *Proc Natl Acad Sci USA.* 1999;96:4569-4574.

112. Taylor HL. Effects of bed rest on cardiovascular function and work performance. *J Appl Physiol.* 1949;2:223-239.

113. Teske JA, Kotz CM. Effect of acute and chronic caloric restriction and metabolic glucoprivation on spontaneous physical activity in obesity-prone and obesity-resistant rats. *Am J Physiol Regul Integr Comp Physiol.* 2009;297:R176-R184.

114. Thivel D, Aucouturier J, Doucet E, Saunders TJ, Chaput J-P. Daily energy balance in children and adolescents. Does energy expenditure predict subsequent energy intake? *Appetite.* 2013;60(1):58-64.

115. Tou JCL, Wade CE. Determinants affecting physical activity levels in animal models. *Exp Biol Med.* 2002;227:587-600.

116. Tremblay A, Cote J, LeBlanc J. Diminished dietary thermogenesis in exercise-trained human subjects. *Eur J Appl Physiol.* 1983;52:1-4.

117. Tremblay A, Fontaine E, Poehlman ET, Mitchell D, Perron L, Bouchard C. The effect of exercise training on resting metabolic rate in lean and moderately obese individuals. *Int J Obes.* 1986;10:511-517.

118. Tremblay A, Nadeau A, Fournier G, Bouchard C. Effect of a three day interruption of exercise training on resting metabolic rate and glucose-induced thermogenesis in trained individuals. *Int J Obes.* 1988;12:163-168.

119. Van Pelt RE, Dinneno FA, Seals DR, Jones PP. Age-related decline in RMR in physically active men: Relation to exercise volume and energy intake. *Am J Physiol Endocrinol Metab.* 2001;281:E633-E639.

120. Van Zant RS. Influence of diet and exercise on energy expenditure. *Int J Sports Nutr.* 1992;2:1-19.

121. Wang Z, O'Connor TP, Heshka S, Heymsfield SB. The reconstruction of Kleiber's law at the organ tissue level. *J Nutr.* 2001;131:2967-2970.

122. West BJ. *Where Medicine Went Wrong. Rediscovering the Path to Complexity.* Singapore: World Scientific; 2006: 37-68.

123. Westerterp KR. Metabolic adaptations to over- and under feeding—still a matter of debate? *Eur J Clin Nutr.* 2013;67:443-445.

124. Westerterp KR, Meijer GA, Janssen EM, Saris WH, Ten Hoof F. Long-term effect of physical activity on energy balance and body composition. *Br J Nutr.* 1992;68:21-30.
125. Wilkin T. Can we modulate physical activity in children? No. *Int J Obes.* 2011;35:1270-1276.
126. Wilterdink EJ, Ballor DL, Keesey RE. Changes in body composition and daily energy expenditure induced in rats during eight weeks of daily swim training. *Int J Obes Rel Metab Disord.* 1993;17:139-143.
127. Woods SC, D'Alessio DA. Central control of body weight and appetite. *J Clin Endocrinol Metab.* 2008;93(Suppl):S37-S50.
128. Zhen H, Lenard N, Shin A, Berthoud H-R. Appetite control and energy balance regulation in the modern world: Reward-driven brain overrides repletion signals. *Int J Obes.* 2009;33(Suppl 2):S8-S13.

Part III and Epilogue

1. Baggett CD, Stevens J, Catellier DJ, Evenson KR, McMurray RG, He K, Tretuh MS. Compensation or displacement of physical activity in middle school girls: The Trial of Activity for Adolescent Girls. *Int J Obes.* 2010;34:1193-1199.
2. Barja-Fernandez S, Leios R, Casanueva FF, Seoane LM. Drug development strategies for the treatment of obesity: How to ensure efficacy, safety, and sustainable weight loss. *Durg Design Develop Ther.* 2014;8:2391-2400.
3. Barres R, Zierath JR. DNA methylation in metabolic disorders. *Am J Clin Nutr.* 2011;93:897S-900S.
4. Berends HI, Nijlant M, Movig KLL, van Putten MJAM, Jannik MJA, Ijzerman MJ. The clinical use of drugs influencing neurotransmitters in the brain to promote motor recovery after stroke: A systematic review. *Eur J Phys Rehabil Med.* 2009;45:621-630.
5. Bernard C. *An Introduction to the Study of Experimental Medicine.* New York: Dover; 1957:135.
6. Berthoud H-R. Interactions between the "cognitive" and "metabolic" brain in the control of food intake. *Phys Behav.* 2007;91:486-498.
7. Biddle SJH, Braithwaite R, Person N. The effectiveness of interventions to increase physical activity among young girls: A meta-analysis. *Prev Med.* 2014;62:119-131.
8. Blundell JE, King NA. Physical activity and regulation of food intake: Current evidence. *Med Sci Sports Exerc.* 1999;31(Suppl 11):S573-S583.
9. Blundell JE, Stubbs RJ, Hughes DA, Whybrow S, King NA. Cross talk between physical activity and appetite control: Does physical activity stimulate appetite? *Proc Nutr Soc.* 2003;62:651-661.

10. Boland CL, Harris JB, Harris KB. Pharmacologic management of obesity for pediatric patients. *Ann Pharmacother.* 2015;49(2): 220-232.

11. Borer KT. Nonhomeostatic control of human appetite and physical activity in regulation of energy balance. *Exerc Sport Sci Rev.* 2010;38:114-121.

12. Bouchard C, Blair SN. Roundtable introduction. Introductory comments for the consensus on physical activity and obesity. *Med Sci Sports Exerc.* 1999;31(Suppl 11);S498-S501.

13. Brown LK. Can sleep deprivation studies explain why human adults sleep? *Curr Opin Pulm Med.* 2012;18(6):541-545.

14. Campbell J. *Myths to Live By.* London: Souvenir Press; 1973.

15. Castañeda TR, Jurgens H, Weidmer P. Obesity and the neuroendocrine control of energy homeostasis: The role of spontaneous locomotor activity. *J Nutr.* 2005;135:1314-1319.

16. Ceccarini G, Maffei M, Vitti P, Santini F. Fuel homeostasis and locomotor behavior: Role of leptin and melanocortin pathways. *J Endocrin Invest.* 2015;38(2):125-131.

17. Chase JA, et al. Interventions to increase physical activity among older adults: A meta-analysis. *Gerontologist.* 2015;55(4):706-718.

18. Clark AM, Clarke ADB. *Early Exposure: Myths and Evidence.* London: Open Books; 1976.

19. Craver CF, Darden L. *In Search of Mechanisms. Discoveries Across the Life Sciences.* Chicago: University of Chicago Press; 2013.

20. Cropper WH. *Great Physicists.* Oxford: Oxford University Press; 2001: 78-105.

21. Dale D, Corbin CB, Dale KS. Restricting opportunities to be active during school time: Do children compensate by increasing physical activity levels after school? *Res Q Exerc Sport.* 2000;71:240-248.

22. Donnelly JE, Hermann SD, Lambourne K, Szabo AN, Honas JJ, Washburn RA. Does increased exercise or physical activity alter ad-libitum energy intake or macronutrient composition in health adults? A systematic review. *PLoS ONE.* 2014;9(1):e83498.

23. Finelli C, Gioia S, La Sala N. Physical activity: An important adaptive mechanism for body weight control. *ISNR Obesity.* 2012; doi:10.5402/2012/675285.

24. Gomersall SR, Rowlands AV, English C, Maher C, Olds TS. The ActivityStat hypothesis: The concept, the evidence and the methodologies. *Sports Med.* 2013;43:135-149.

25. Goodman A, Mackett RL, Paskins J. Activity compensation and activity synergy in British 8-13 year olds. *Prev Med.* 2011;53(4-5):293-298.

26. Gopnik A. Mindless. The new neuro-skeptics. *The New Yorker.* September 9, 2013: 86-88.

27. Goran MI, Poehlman ET. Endurance training does not enhance total energy expenditure in healthy elderly persons. *Am J Physiol.* 1992;263:E950-E957.

28. Hall KD, Heymsfield SB, Kemnitz JW, Kelin S, Schoeller DA, Speakman JR. Energy balance and its components: Implications for body weight regulation. *Am J Clin Nutr.* 2012;95:989-995.

29. Hay J. Activity measurement: Not simply child's play. *Pediatr Exerc Science.* 2013;25:536-547.

30. Heath GW, Parra DC, Sarmiento OL. Evidence-based intervention in physical activity: Lessons from around the world. *Lancet.* 2012;380:272-281.

31. Herrera BM, Keildson S, Lindgren CM. Genetics and epigenetics of obesity. *Maturitas.* 2011;69:41-49.

32. Hobbs N, Godfrey A, Lara J, Errington L, Meyer TD, Rochester L, White M, et al. Are behavioral interventions effective in increasing physical activity at 12 to 36 months in adults aged 55 to 70 years? A systematic review and meta-analysis. *BMC Medicine.* 2013;11:75.

33. Keesey RE, Hirvonen MD. Body weight set-points: Determination and adjustment. *J Nutr.* 1997;127:1875S-1883S.

34. Kimm SYS, Glynn NW, Kriska AM, Barton BA, Kronsberg SS, Daniels SR, Crawford PB, et al. Decline in physical activity in black girls and white girls during adolescence. *N Engl J Med.* 2002;347:709-715.

35. King NA. The relationship between physical activity and food intake. *Proc Nutr Soc.* 1998;57:1-9.

36. King NA, Caudwell P, Hopkins M, Byrne NM, Colley RC, Hills AP, Stubbs, JR, et al. Metabolic and behavioral compensatory responses to exercise interventions: Barriers to weight loss. *Obesity.* 2007;15:1373-1383.

37. Kleim JA, Jones TA, Schallert T. Motor enrichment and the induction of plasticity before or after brain injury. *Neurochem Res.* 2003;28:1757-1769.

38. Krol E, Duncan JS, Redman P, Morgan PJ, Mercer JG, Speakman JR. Photoperiod regulates leptin sensitivity in field voles, *Microtus agrestis. J Com Physiol B Biochem Sys Environ.* 2006;176:153-163.

39. Levine JA. Non-exercise activity thermogenesis. *Proc Nutr Soc.* 2003;62:667-679.

40. Levine JA, Kotz CM. NEAT—non-exercise activity thermogenesis—egocentric & geocentric environmental factors vs. biological regulation. *Acta Physiol Scand.* 2005;184:309-318.

41. Levine JA, Eberhardt NL, Jensen MD. Role of nonexercise activity thermogenesis in resistance to fat gain in humans. *Science.* 1999;283:212-214.
42. Lore RK. Activity-drive hypothesis: Effects of activity restriction. *Psych Bull.* 1968;70:566-574.
43. Lorenz K. *Behind the Mirror. A Search for a Natural History of Human Knowledge.* London: Methuen; 1977.
44. Matsuda M, Liu Y, Mahankali S, Pu Y, Mahandali A, Wang J, DeFronzo RA, et al. Altered hypothalamic function in response to glucose ingestion in obese humans. *Diabetes.* 1999;48:1801-1806.
45. Mayer J, Roy P, Mitra KP. Relation between caloric intake, body weight, and physical work: Studies in an industrial male population in West Bengal. *Am J Clin Nutr.* 1956;4:169-175.
46. McAllister EJ, Dhurandhar NV, Keith SW, Aronne LJ, Barger J, Baskin M, Benca RM, et al. Ten putative contributors to the obesity epidemic. *Crit Rev Food Sci Nutr.* 2009;49:868-913.
47. Metcalf B, Henley W, Wilkin T. Effectiveness of intervention on physical activity of children: Systematic review and meta-analysis of controlled trials with objectively measured outcomes (Early Bird 54). *BMJ.* 2012;345:e5888.
48. Pearson N, Braithwaite R, Biddle SJ. The effectiveness of interventions to increase physical activity among adolescent girls: A meta-analysis. *Acad Pediatr.* 2015;15:9-18.
49. Plachta-Danielzik S, Landsberg B, Bosy-Westphal A. Energy gain and energy gap in normal-weight children: Longitudinal data of the KOPS. *Obesity.* 2008;16:777-783.
50. Ponjee GA, Janssen EM, Hermans J, van Wersch JW. Effects of long-term exercise of moderate intensity on anthropometric values and serum lipids and lipoproteins. *Eur J Clin Chem Clin Biochem.* 1995;33:121-126.
51. Poudel GR, Innes CRH, Bones PJ, Watts R, Jones RD. Losing the struggle to stay awake: Divergent thalamic and cortical activity during microsleeps. *Hum Brain Map.* 2014;35:257-269.
52. Ravussin E, Bogardus C. Energy balance and weight regulation: Genetics versus environment. *Br J Nutr.* 2000;83(Suppl 1):S17-S20.
53. Ravussin E, Lillioja S, Anderson TE, Christin L, Bogardus C. Determinants of 24-hour energy expenditure in man. *J Clin Invest.* 1986;78:1568-1578.
54. Rechtschaffen A, Bergmann BM, Everson CA, Kushida CA, Billiland MA. Sleep deprivation in the rat. X. Integration and discussion of findings. *Sleep.* 2002;25:68-87.

55. Reilly JJ. Can we modulate physical activity in children? *Int J Obes.* 2011;35:1266-1269.

56. Ridgers ND, Timperio A, Cerin E, Salmon J. Compensation of physical activity and sedentary time in primary school children. *Med Sci Sports Exerc.* 2014;46:1564-1569.

57. Rosner MH. Exercise-associated hyponatremia. *Semin Nephrol.* 2009;29:271-281.

58. Rowland T. The childhood obesity epidemic: Putting the "dynamics" into thermodynamics. *Pediatr Exerc Science.* 2004;16:87-93.

59. Rowland T. Promoting physical activity for children's health. Rationale and strategies. *Sports Med.* 2007;37:929-936.

60. Rowland T. On Lamarck, lima beans, and learning of physical activity habits. *Pediatr Exerc Science.* 2008;20:1-4.

61. Rowland T. *The Athlete's Clock.* Champaign, IL: Human Kinetics; 2011: 8-17.

62. Rowlands AV. Methodological approaches for investigating the biological basis for physical activity in children. *Pediatr Exerc Science.* 2009;21:273-278.

63. Saris WHM, van Erp-Baart MA, Browns F, Westerterp KR, ten Hoor F. Study on food intake and energy expenditure during extreme sustained exercise: The Tour de France. *Int J Sports Med.* 1989;10: S26-S31.

64. Schoeller DA. The energy balance equation: Looking back and looking forward are two very different views. *Nutr Rev.* 2009;67:249-254.

65. Shaibi GQ, Ryder JR, Kim JY, Barraza E. Exercise for obese youth: Refocusing attention from weight loss to health gains. *Exerc Sport Sci Rev.* 2015;43:41-47.

66. Shephard RJ, Jequier J-C, Lavallee H, LaBarre R, Rajic M. Habitual physical activity: Effects of sex, milieu, season and required activity. *J Sports Med.* 1980;20:55-66.

67. Sluckin W. *Early Learning in Man and Animal.* London: George Allen and Unwin; 1970.

68. Speelman AD, van de Warrenburg BP, van Nimwegen M, Petzinger GM, Munneke M, Bloem BR. How might physical activity benefit patients with Parkinson disease? *Nat Rev Neurol.* 2011;7: 528-534.

69. Storey KB, Storey JM. Metabolic rate depression and biochemical adaptation in anaerobiosis, hibernation and estivation. *Quart Rev Biol.* 1990;65:145-165.

70. Telama R. Tracking of physical activity from childhood to adulthood: A review. *Obes Facts.* 2009;3:187-195.

71. Thivel D, Aucouturier J, Doucet E, Saunders TJ, Chaput J-P. Daily energy balance in children and adolescents. Does energy expenditure predict subsequent energy intake? *Appetite.* 2013;60:58-64.
72. Thorburn AW, Proietto J. Biological determinants of spontaneous physical activity. *Obes Rev.* 2000;1:87-94.
73. U.S. Department of Health and Human Services. Physical activity and health: A report of the Surgeon General. Atlanta, GA: U.S. Department of Health and Human Services, Centers for Disease Control and Prevention. National Center for Chronic Disease Prevention and Health Promotion; 1996.
74. Van Vliet-Ostaptchouk, Sneider H, Lagou V. Gene-lifestyle interactions in obesity. *Curr Nutr Rep.* 2012;1:184-196.
75. Van Sluijs EMF, McMinn AM, Griffin SJ. Effectiveness of interventions to promote physical activity in children and adolescents: Systematic review of controlled trials. *Brit Med J.* 2008;42(8):653-657.
76. Waterland RA, Jirtle RL. Early nutrition, epigenetic changes at transposons and imprinted genes, and enhanced susceptibility to adult chronic disease. *Nutrition.* 2004;20(1):63-68.
77. Wilkin TJ. Can we modulate physical activity in children? No. *Int J Obes.* 2011;35:1270-1276.
78. Wilkin TJ, Mallam KM, Metcalf BS, Jeffery AN, Voss LD. Variation in physical activity lies with the child, not his environment: Evidence for an 'activitystat' in young children (EarlyBird 16). *Int J Obes.* 2006;30(7):1050-1055.
79. Yanovski SZ, Yanovsky JA. Long-term drug treatment for obesity: A systematic and clinical review. *JAMA.* 2014;311:74-86.
80. Zheng H, Lenard N, Shin A, Berthoud H-R. Appetite control and energy balance regulation in the modern world: Reward-driven brain overrides repletion signals. *Int J Obes.* 2009;33(Suppl 2):S8-S13.
81. Zurlo F, Ferraro RT, Fontvieille AM, Rising R, Bogardus C, Ravussin E. Spontaneous physical activity and obesity: Cross-sectional and longitudinal studies in Pima Indians. *Am J Physiol.* 1992;263:E296-E300.

Index

Note: Page references followed by an italicized *f* or *t* indicate information contained in figures or tables, respectively.

About the Author

Thomas W. Rowland, MD, is a pediatric cardiologist at the Baystate Medical Center in Springfield, Massachusetts. He is a professor of pediatrics at Tufts University School of Medicine and was a past adjunct professor of exercise science at the University of Massachusetts at Amherst. A graduate of the University of Michigan Medical School, Rowland is board certified in pediatrics and pediatric cardiology by the American Board of Pediatrics.

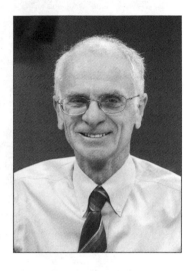

Rowland, who has had more than 150 journal articles published, is the author of three books: *Children's Exercise Physiology, Second Edition; Tennisology: Inside the Science of Serves, Nerves, and On-Court Dominance;* and *The Athlete's Clock.* He has served as editor of the journal *Pediatric Exercise Science* and president of the North American Society for Pediatric Exercise Medicine (NASPEM) and was on the board of trustees of the American College of Sports Medicine (ACSM). He is past president of the New England chapter of the ACSM and received the ACSM Honor Award in 1993.

Rowland is a competitive tennis player and distance runner. He and his wife, Margot, reside in Longmeadow, Massachusetts.

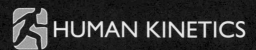
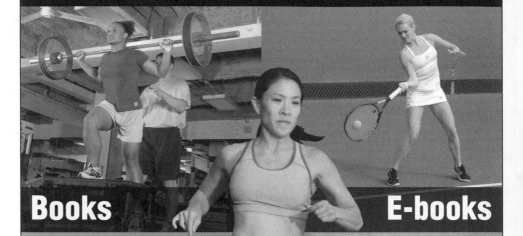